M.O.M's OSCEs
and practical tricks

INTERNATIONAL EDITION - 2021

INTERNATIONAL EDITION
2021

M.O.M's OSCEs
and practical tricks

THE 1st BOOK FROM M.A.S & M.O.M SERIES

Edited by:
Mohammed I. al-Musawi, M.B.Ch.B (College of Medicine University of Baghdad -2012)

Revision by:
Mohammed A. al-Saffar, M.B.Ch.B (College of Medicine University of Baghdad -2012)

Haider Salam al-Shiwily, M.B.Ch.B (College of Medicine University of Baghdad -2012)

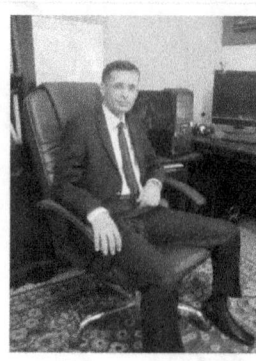

Mohammed Imran Hadi al-Musawi
(Dr. M.O.M.)

Graduated from:
College of Medicine, University of Baghdad
2011 – 2012

** This picture in my dear friend ' Dr. Ahmed Jwad al-Qassam ' home..

Dedication :
  To my wife , *Zainab*

CONTENTS

iii & iv - PREFACE
v & vi - ACKNOWLEDGMENT

1- MEDICINE

HISTORY TAKING	2
HISTORY CASE SHEET	4
CARDIOVASCULAR SYSTEM	
General E_x	4
Precordium E_x	16
Auscultation of precordium	17
Radial pulse E_x	17
JVP E_x	17
Heart sounds & murmurs	18
RESPIRATORY SYSTEM	
General E_x	19
Chest E_x	20
Chest examination from the back	21
GASTROINTESTINAL	
General E_x	22
Abdomen E_x	23
GENERAL EXAMINATION	25
HAND & WRIST EXAMINATION	26
NERVOUS SYSTEM	
General E_x	27
Cranial nerves E_x	29
Upper limb motor E_x	32
Lower limb motor E_x	33
Coordination	34
Sensory E_x	34
Hand nerve supply E_x	35

2- ECG by Dr. M.O.M

INTRODUCTION	38
WAVES & INTERVALS	42
CARDIAC AXIS	46
HYPERTROPHY	48
ISCHEMIC HEART DISEASE	49
HEART BLOCK	51
DYSARRHYTHMIA	53
HYPE- & HYPO-KALEMIA	56
PERICARDITIS VS. INFARCTION	57
HOW TO READ & REPORT ECG	58
OTHER TOPICS	59

3- SURGERY

HISTORY TAKING	
Pain H_x	62
Yellowish discoloration of sclera & skin H_x	63
Bleeding per rectum H_x	64
Lump or Ulcer H_x	65
Goiter H_x	66
Breast lump H_x	67
Peptic ulcer H_x	68
Upper gastrointestinal bleeding H_x	69
Gallstone pain H_x	70
Gastric outlet obstruction H_x	70
EXAMINATION	
Ulcer E_x	71
Lump E_x	72
Thyroid status E_x	73
Thyroid E_x	74
Hernia E_x	75
Breast E_x	77
Abdominal E_x	78
Post-operative E_x	79
Wound E_x	80
Chest tube E_x	81
Drains E_x	82
Stoma E_x	83
PERIPHERAL VASCULAR EXAMINATION	
Lower limb	84
Varicose veins	86
Upper limb	87
MEDICAL SKILL LAB	
Per rectum examination	89
Nasogastric tube placement	90
Foley's catheter insertion	91
Cannula insertion	92
Chest tube placement	93
I.M. injection	94
Indications, complications, C.I...etc	95
RADIOLOGY	
How to report 'Chest X-ray'	97
How to report 'Abdominal X-ray'	98
Some of important X-rays & other radiological studies	99
UROSURGERY	
Genitourinary problems 'H$_x$ taking'	101
Hematuria H_x, pain H_x	102
Abdominal E_x	103
General E_x related to urosurgery	103
Genital E_x	105
How to report 'urosurgery radiological studies'	106
Urosurgery - Instruments	108

4- ORTHOPEDICS

EXAMINATION	
Shoulder joint	112
Elbow joint	114
Hip joint	116
Knee joint	118

i

CONTENTS

Wrist & hand	120
Ankle joint & foot	122
Back (Lumbar spine)	124
Neck (Cervical spine)	126
HOW TO REPORT ' The orthopedics & fracture X-ray '	128

5- PEDIATRICS

HISTORY TAKING

CASE SHEET	131
Jaundice H_x	136
Hematuria	137
Fit H_x	138
Enuresis H_x	139
Joint swelling H_x	140
Diabetes mellitus H_x	141
Diarrhea H_x	142
Wheezy chest H_x	143
Cough H_x	144
Fever H_x	145
Cardiac disease H_x	146

EXAMINATION

General Ex	147
Respiratory distress Assessment	148
Hydration status assessment	148
Nutritional status assessment	149
Patient with meningitis	150
Patient with bleeding tendency	151
Patient with diabetes	152
Patient with jaundice	153
Patient with Hematuria	154
Patient with diarrhea	154
Patient with edema (N.S.)	155
Patient with hydrocephalus	156
Patient with rickets	156
Down syndrome	157
Temperature measurement	157
Height measurement in children	158

COMMUNICATION SKILLS

Diabetes mellitus ' Insulin injection '	159
Diabetes mellitus ' Diabetes diet '	160
Diabetes M. ' Hypoglycemic attacks '	160
D. M. ' How to use a glucometer '	161
Lumbar puncture	162
Breast feeding	164
Oral rehydration solution (O.R.S.)	165
Enuresis	166
Vaccinations	167
Vaccines	169

INVESTIGATIONS

Normal values	171
C.S.F. analysis	172
N. S. vs. Glumerilunephritis	173
Trick - Hematology	174
FOLLOW UP CHARTS	175
DEVELOPMENT MADE VERY EASY	176
DRUGs ' ESSENTIAL NOTEs '	178
INTRAVENOUS FLUIDs	187
BLOOD PRODUCTs	189

OTHER IMPORTANT TOPICS

Lumbar puncture	190
Bone marrow aspiration & biopsy	190
Exchange transfusion	191
Phototherapy	192
Ventolin nubulizar (Salbutamol)	192
Different types of drips	193
Intraousseous needle	193
Liver biopsy	194
Urine analysis (Urine dipstick)	194
Other important topics	194

6- GYNECOLOGY & OBSTETRICS

H_x CASE SHEET	196

EXAMINATION

Obstetric abdominal E_x	200
Gynecological P.V. E_x	202
Clinical pelvimetry	203
Post-operative assessment	204
PARTOGRAM	205
FORCEPS & INSTRUMENTS	212
OXYTOCIN & METHERGINE	223

iii – PREFACE of the FIRST EDITION

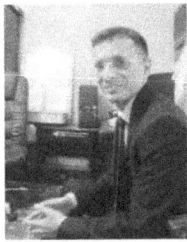

During my studies in the 4th grade in the Faculty of Medicine, University of Baghdad, I had some difficulties to remember some of important steps (with my knowledge of the correct way to do it) during examination, like I always forget to do the liver span in abdominal examination or to do vocal resonance in the chest E_x..etc '..

So, I thought of a possible way in which I can arrange these steps to avoid these mistakes..

I started to summarize the steps of medical history taking and clinical examination in a way that is easy to remember and I continued with this approach in subsequent years and in all medical branches (Medicine, Surgery, Pediatric & Gynecology and Obstetrics)..

In 6th grade, I realized that what I have done previously was of great value through the great benefits that I got, especially in the final exams, because the summaries were short and do not require a long time to read, in addition to relying on valuable references like (Macleod's clinical examination, BROWSE, Apleys System of Orthopaedics and Fractures & TEN Teachers..etc) and also on the sessions notes & our lectures in the college..

And after I finished the final exams, I saw that what I wrote could be a beneficial book for all my fellow students.. So, I decided to write this book, hoping to be a source of knowledge that all students can rely on..

This book consists of 6 chapters, and is designed to be every page is a one OSCE ' *Objective Structured Clinical Examination* ' station (or more) & I have alluded to some of the tricks that despite its simplicity it is of great importance during the practical practice..

I've deleted all the question marks (?) and question formats and some words that are understandable within the context of the text

(for example: I am looking for scar, stria..etc)..

And I have depending on the colors to signify some meanings, as following:

Headlines..	Less important..
Sub-divisions..	Not so important..
Very important..	Forget it..
Important..	Text (in general)..

I mentioned in this book the purely practical practice (although I mentioned some theoretical points that are part of the OSCE stations).. But, you can read all the techniques & all the theoretical topics in your textbooks, lectures, session notes, tutorial & the supported DVDs with this book..

Finally, this book is intended for students in the 6th grade (Stagers) in particular ' *but this does not mean that it isn't beneficial to students in other grades, particularly the 4th grade of the Faculty of Medicine* ', and this book is not considered as an alternative to the important references but it is consider as a short, rapid and concentrated summery for these references.. Perhaps that offers even the little thing for the student and permeated interest to everyone..

Mohammed Imran al-Musawi
' M.O.M. ' 2021

iv – PREFACE of THE 2nd EDITION

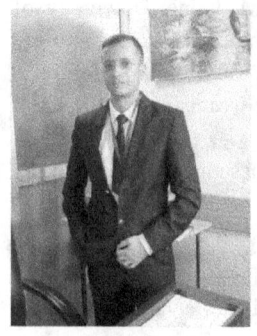

I believe that the main object of basic medical education is to train the student to talk to and to examine a patient, in such a way that he can discover the full history of the patient's illness and elicit the abnormal physical signs to reach a differential diagnosis and suggest likely methods of treatment ..

In this edition, I have attempted to describe *THE STEPs* in History taking and in Physical examination .. so, I mention a history **CASE SHEETs** of many medical branches and I review all the chapters in this book, and add some OSCE stations that make this book one of the most important resources in HISTORY TAKING and OSCEs Stations.

I hope this book will be more of a **teaching book** than just a text-book, which will be read many times during your basic and higher medical training ..

The continuing success of this book indicate that it helps to fill the deficit that exist in the other books.. *So, enjoy with this book..*

God bless you..

Dr. Mohammed Imran al-Musawi
' Dr. M.O.M. ' 2021

v - ACKNOWLEDGMENTS

I am very grateful to my friends Dr. Haider Abdulkareem Qasim & Dr. Mohammed Kadhim Al-Hashimi for their invaluable help & support especially in the 6th grade in medical college and ***all my real friends*** '& especially to mention, Dr. Ahmed Jwad al-Qassam, Dr. Mryiam Issa al-Ani, Dr. Juhayna Kefah Abd-al Wahaab, & Dr. Ahmed Kifah al-Esamy'.. *also, I would like to thank my wife & family for their encouragement & for everything they have done for me during my university studies & in all my life..*

I think it is important to thank the admins & members of the "OSCE group" on Facebook, for their great helping hands in our success..

And the last but not least, this book would not have been possible without the help of ALL OUR DOCTORs who have long worked hard to teach us during the past six years..

Dr. Mohammed Imran al-Musawi
' M.O.M. ' 2012 - 2013

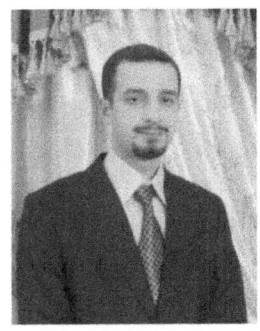

In every human life there is frustration & there is success, but only those who can challenge would change their fate & struggle for the success no matter how long it could take… we present this book to you hoping for the best that you can make by understanding the notes & tricks, so as to overcome the difficulties that you may face in every aspect in your clinical rounds & OSCE exams…

I would like to thank my sisters *Dr. Fatima & Dr. Zahra A. al-Saffar* (from Al-Nahrain medical college)… & my best friends for their support…

Dr. Mohammed Abdulredha al-Saffar
MAS - 2012

vi - SPECIAL ACKNOWLEDGMENTS

This book would not have been possible without the help of the my friend Dr. Haider Salam al-Shiwily ..

GOD BLESS YOU ..

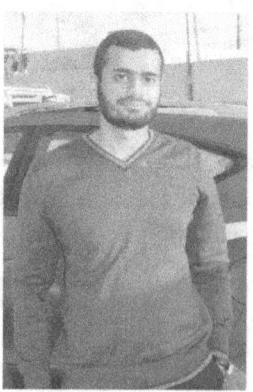

CHAPTER 1

MEDICINE

Contents:

HISTORY TAKING	2
HISTORY CASE SHEETs	4
CARDIOVASCULAR SYSTEM	
General E_x	15
Precordium E_x	16
Auscultation of precordium	17
Radial pulse E_x	17
JVP E_x	17
Heart sounds & murmurs	18
RESPIRATORY SYSTEM	
General E_x	19
Chest E_x	20
Chest examination from the back	21
GASTROINTESTINAL	
General E_x	22
Abdomen E_x	23
GENERAL EXAMINATION	25
HAND & WRIST E_x	26
NERVOUS SYSTEM	
General E_x	27
Cranial nerves E_x	29
Upper limb motor E_x	32
Lower limb motor E_x	33
Coordination	34
Sensory E_x	34
Hand nerve supply E_x	35

1- MEDICINE — HISTORY TAKING..

The art of History Taking and Report:

There are many books that talk in details about the history taking, but I want to explain it in a way entirely different and touch some of the important points that must be observed to improve your skill in History Taking and Report..

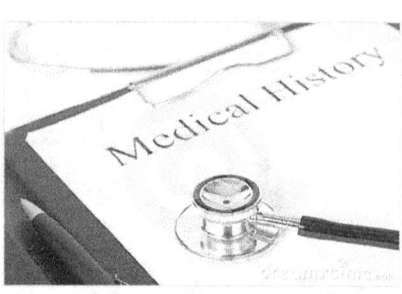
www.webdicine.com

The history case sheet, in general, can be divided into 5 parts:
- demography
- chief complaint and duration
- history of present illness
- review of systems
- past medical H_x, past surgical H_x, drug H_x, family H_x, socioeconomic H_x & occupational H_x

---

HISTORY CASE SHEET:

Name: Ahmed Mohammed Aziz
Age: 45 years old
Sex: male
Address: al-sha'ab/Baghdad
Occupation: policeman
Religion: muslim
Marital state: married
Date of admission: 21/1/2012
Date of taking H_x: 23/1/2012

→ Demography..

Source of information: the patient himself (no need for mention it, if the H. was from the patient)

Chief complaint & duration: shortness of breath for 3 hours

H_x of present illness: → Trick: start with the 1st time that he feel unwell even it was before many years. Continue till you reach the chief complaint & mention all it's details and complete the details of the system involved, then the details of his condition in the hospital.
You can mention for example "the patient is a known case of diabetes mellitus since 3 years, good controlled, on diet & daonil 5 mg/d" at the bigining.

Review of systems:
Past medical H_x:
Past surgical H_x:
Drug H_x:
Family H_x:
Socioeconomic H_x:
Occupational H_x:

Trick: Don't repeat the system that mentioned in the history of present illness & start with most relevant system to the system involved.

1- MEDICINE — HISTORY TAKING..

★★ Now, the BIG question is ' *HOW TO REPORT THE HISTORY ??* '

The answer is ' *Report it like a STORY* ' & please, *FORGET* the divisions of the history case sheet..

~~Name, Age, Sex, Chief Complaint, H_x of present~~ illness...... etc.

So, the reporting of previous examples is:

I would like to present my case.. Whose name is Ahmed Mohammed Aziz, he is 45 years old, male, living in al-sha'ab / Baghdad & he is muslim, married, work as a policeman, admitted into hospital on twenty first of January 2012, I 'am taking the history on twenty third of January 2012.

The patient presented with shortness of breath for 3 hours, the condition started as a dry cough before 2 week ………………………………….. etc.

★★ The history differs from one department to another; like in pediatric 'for example' concentrates on natal H_x, vaccination, developmental and other divisions which are not present in the history of MEDICINE and so on.. BUT, the idea in *History Taking and Report* is the same.

Trick: NEVER EVER repeat any symptom, You mentioned it previously in the H. ...
Ex. When you mention the Chest Pain in the H_x of present illness .. Don't mention it again in the Respiratory system, and so on ...

1- MEDICINE — HISTORY TAKING [CASE SHEET]..

HISTORY CASE SHEET :

DEMOGRAPHIC DATA OF THE PATIENT :

Name:
Age :
Sex :
Address :
Occupation :
Religion :
Marital status :
Date of admission to hospital :
Date of taking history :
Source of information (The patient himself or a relative ?) :

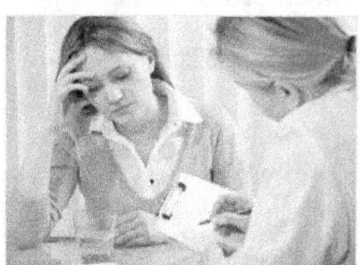
www.crop-doctor-patient.com

CHIEF COMPLAINT & DURATION:

> Ex. Shortness of breath for 4 days prior to admission
> Abdominal pain for 6 hours prior to admission

H. OF PRESENT ILLNESS.

Tell me about your complaint(s) in details & from the beginning .. !!

How and when the illness started (SYSTEM INVOLVED) ?

Any changes in the course of the illness ?

Any drugs are given ? any benefit ?

Mention the effect of illness on :

- Appetite ?
- Weight ?
- Bowel motion ?
- Urine output ?
- Sleep ?
- Activity ?

Progress of illness in the hospital ?

Any pain ? [PAIN ANALYSIS]

Any INCREASE IN BODY TEMPERATURE ?

1- MEDICINE — HISTORY TAKING [CASE SHEET]..

PAIN ANALYSIS :

' You have to ask about all these questions , whenever the patient tell you he has pain anywhere in the body !!! '

Exact site ?
Duration ?
Character ?
Onset ? *(suddenly or gradually started)*
Radiation ?
Severity ?
Frequency ?
Aggravating factors ?
Relieving factors ?
Associated symptoms ?

INCREASED BODY TEMPERATURE :

' You have to ask about all these questions , whenever the patient tell you he has increase in body temperature !!! '

Onset ?
Duration ?
Grade ?
Continuous , Intermittent or Remittent ?
Constant or Progressive ?
Associated with sweating (mild or drenching sweating) , Chills or Rigor ?
At day time or at night ?
Relieve by cool sponging or medication ?
Associated symptoms ?

SYSTEMS REVIEW :

ALIMENTARY SYSTEM & THE ABDOMEN :

Condition of the mouth : Ulcers ? , Pain ? , Lost teeth ? , Dry mouth , Abnormal taste ?

Difficulty in swallowing : For liquids or with solid food ? , painful swallowing ? , Food stuck ? Level ?

Regurgitation : *' Is effortless return of food into the mouth '*
What comes up .. liquid or food ?
How often does it occur ?
Precipitating factors ? ex. Straining ..

Nausea : Associated with or followed by vomiting ?

1- MEDICINE — HISTORY TAKING [CASE SHEET]..

Vomiting : Frequency ?
Relating to meal-time?
Quantity ?
Contents & Color ?: Recognizable food from previous meal ? ,
Digested food ? ,
Bile stained fluid ? ,
Feculent ?
Contain blood or Coffee ground ?
Relation of vomiting to pain ? Does it relieve pain ?
Effortful or effortless (projectile) ?
Preceded by another symptom such as headache or pain ?
Early morning vomiting?
Precipitating or relieving factors ?

Heart burn : *' Pain behind the sternum '*
Frequency ?
Come-on on lying down ?
Precipitating factors ?

Water brush : *' Excessive secretion of saliva '*

Flatulence : Relieve the symptoms ?

Abdominal pain : [Pain analysis..]
Relation to meal ?
Relieve by defecation or by passage of flatus ?

Abdominal distension : What brought this to his attention ?
When did it begin & how has it progress ?
Painful ?
Affect respiration ?
Relieved by belching , vomiting or defecation ?

Constipation : Frequency ? (Motion / Day)
Your usual bowel habit ?
Any recent change in habit ?
Any change in diet or medication ?
Does the constipation alternate with diarrhea ?
Any colicky pain ?
Any blood in the stool ?

1- MEDICINE — HISTORY TAKING [CASE SHEET]..

NATURE OF THE STOOL :
- Color : brown , black , white or silver ?
- Consistence : hard , soft or watery ?
- Size : bulky , pellets or tape like ?
- Does it float on water on sink ?
- Smell ?
- Mixed with mucus ?
- Anal itching ?
- Any dark tarry stool ' *it is called melena* & *it indicates upper GIT bleeding* '

***Frequent bowel motion** 'Diarrhea'* :
- Frequency (motion / day) ?
- Usual bowel motion ?
- Relation to meal ?
- Painful defecation ?
- Purgative use ?
- Incontinence to formed stool ?
- Do you drink clean tap water ?
- NATURE OF STOOL ? *(Mentioned previously)*..

Yellowish discoloration of the conjunctiva or skin :
- Onset ?
- Duration ?
- Tea color urine ?
- Pale or dark bowel motion ?
- Skin itching ?
- Any case of jaundice among family , friends or work-mates ?
- H_x of blood transfusion ?
- H_x of drinking alcohol ?
- H_x of travelling abroad recently ?
- H_x of any kind of injection in the last 3 – 4 months ?
- Any abdominal pain ?

Appetite & Weight :
- Increased or decreased ?
- Does the size of your T shirt or shoes is not suitable to you , now ?

1- MEDICINE — HISTORY TAKING [CASE SHEET]..

RESPIRATORY SYSTEM :

Cough : Dry or productive ?
  Worse at specific time of day ?
  Come in episode ?
  Duration ?
  Worse by particular condition such as cold or dust ?
  Painful ?
  Chocking or blush discoloration of the face , lips or limbs ?

Sputum : How much ?
  Most produce at particular time of day or at night ??
  Consistency ?
  Color ?
  Odor ?
  Blood stained ? *(Streaks or clots ? , On how many occasions ?)*
  Purulent ?

Shortness of breath : Duration ?
  Onset ?
  At rest , after exertion ? or after walking (distance ?)

Wheeze : Constant or intermitted ?
  Anything provoke it ?
  Worse at particular time of day or at night ?

Chest pain : [Pain analysis..]
  Aggravated by deep breathing or coughing ?
  Associated with cough , sputum or shortness of breath ?

Hoarseness of voice : Constant or intermitted ?

Bluish discoloration of the face , lips or limbs :

1- MEDICINE — HISTORY TAKING [CASE SHEET]..

CARDIOVASCULAR SYSTEM :

Chest pain : [Pain analysis..]
        Especially.. The exact site ?
                Character ?
                Radiate to *the left arm , neck , shoulder or interscapular region ?*
                On exertion or at rest ?
                Precipitating and relieving factors ?
                Relieved by rest ?

Awareness of heart beats ' Palpitation ' :
        Duration ?
        Induced or relieved by exercise ?
        The heart beats rate is increased ?
        The heart beats are regular or irregular ?
        Do you drink a lot of tea, coffee or alcohol ?
        H_x of sudden death in the family ?

Shortness of breath : Onset ?
                Duration ?
                At rest or on exertion ?
                What degree of exertion is necessary ?
                      (ex. After walking 10 meters)

Shortness of breath on lying flat :
        No. of pillows to breath freely ?
        Relived if he sleep on specific side ?

Shortness of breath in the middle of night :
        Sudden attack that waken the patient ?
        Associated factors ?

Ankle or leg swelling : Duration ?
                Progression ?
                In one leg or both legs ?
                Affected by bed rest &/or elevation of the leg ?
                Any change in skin color ?
                Associated with fatigue in the legs ?

1- MEDICINE
HISTORY TAKING [CASE SHEET]..

Leg pain on exertion: [Pain analysis..]
    Especially.. The exact site ?
        Which muscles are involved ? Which part is painful ?
        How far can he walk before the pain begins ?
        So bad that has to stop walking ?
        How long it take to disappear ?
        Can he walk the same distance again ?
        Any pain at rest ?
        Relieved by analgesic drugs ?
        What position relieve the pain ?
        Cold extremities ?
        Any change in skin color particularly in response to cold ?
        Any numbness or tingling in limbs ?
        Any intermittent claudication ?

UROGENITAL SYSTEM :

Loin pain : [Pain analysis..]
Burning micturition ?
Frequency of micturition ?
Volume of urine ?
Urgent need to urinate ? (After stress ?)
Awake at night to pass urine ?
Color of urine ? , Turbid ?
Any blood ?
Difficulty in starting the stream ? , Poor stream ? , Terminal dribbling ?
Headache , Drowsiness , Fit , Vomiting , Constipation or Visual disturbance ?
Ankles , Leg swellings , Puffy face or any other part of the body ?
Urethral discharge ?
H_x of renal stones ?

in MALE :
  Erection ? , Potency ? , Ejaculation ? , Urethral ulcer ? , Libido ?

in FEMALE :
  Age & nature of onset of menstruation ?
  Regular periods ? , Length of each period ? , Amount of blood loss ?
  Date of last menstrual period ?
  The age of cessation of menstruation ?
  Any blood loss after the days of the periods ?
  No. of pregnancies ?, No. of live births ?
  H_x of prolonged or obstructed labor ?

1- MEDICINE — HISTORY TAKING [CASE SHEET]..

NERVOUS SYSTEM :

Headache : [Pain analysis..]

Tremor : Onset ?
    Continuous or intermitted ?
    At rest , intension or on movement ?

Seizures : First attack ?
    Shortest & longest interval between attacks ?
    Occur during sleep ?
    Any warning symptoms before the attacks ?
    Any Loss of consciousness , Tongue bite or Incontinence ?
    Postictal symptoms like sleep , headache , paralysis or change in behavior ?
    Was the mental state affected ?
    Drug H_x?
    There is any witness to the attack ?

Faint or Blackout : Duration ?
    When did occur ?
    First attack ?
    When & where the patient awake up ?
    Spontaneously or after stimulation by something ?
    Any associated symptoms ?

Tingling or Numbness : Site ?
    Intermitted or continuous ?
    Increase with specific posture ?
    Severity ?

Ankle or leg swelling : Duration ?
    Progression ?
    In one leg or both legs ?
    Affected by bed rest &/or elevation of the leg ?
    Any change in skin color ?
    Associated with fatigue in the legs ?

Stroke : Onset ?
    Duration ?
    Any headache ?
    Any loss of consciousness ?
    Does the symptoms improved with time ?

1- MEDICINE — HISTORY TAKING [CASE SHEET]..

Any incontinence ?
Any weakness or loss of sensation affecting one side or both sides of the body ? Symmetrical ?
Any difficulty in wearing clothes , combing the hair , standing from sitting position , getting upstairs ? *(Proximal muscle weakness)*
Any difficulty in buttoning and unbuttoning his shirts , using keys of the doors ?
Any weakness affecting the muscles of the eye lids , upper limbs & lower limbs ?
Any loss of vision ?
Any hearing problem ? in one side or both sides ?
Any previous attack ?
Past medical H_x of H.T. , D.M. , angina pectoris ?
Smoker ?
Same previous condition in the family ?
Any dizziness ? Increase with particular posture ?
Any H_x of previous injury or viral infection ?

LOCOMOTOR SYSTEM :

Muscles , Bones or Joints pain: [Pain analysis..]

Joint swelling : One joint or multiple joints ?
        Onset & progression ?
        Painful ?
        Loss of motion ?
        The joint get locked ?
        Any movement can't be perfumed ? Why ? When ?
        H_x of gout or hemophilia ?

Weakness : *(Mentioned previously in nervous system)*

Vision : Appearance of the eyes : *Any abnormality ?*
                              How does it started ?
                                Does it affect vision ? How ?
                                Any pain ? [Pain analysis..]

      Disturbance of vision : *Onset & duration ?*
                                  Continuous or intermitted ?
                                  Aggravating & relieving factors ?
                                  Does the patient use glasses ? Why ? When ?

1- MEDICINE
HISTORY TAKING [CASE SHEET]..

ENDOCRINE SYSTEM :

Heat & cold intolerance : In comparison to other members of family or in work ?
Appetite ?
Weight ?
Awareness of heart beats ' Palpitation ' ?
Loss of consciousness ?
Change in the sweating : Any episode of excessive sweating ?
Any eyes prominence ?
Any swelling in the neck ?
Is the salt used by the patient supplemented with iodine ?
Thirst : How much water does he drink ?
  Any increase in the amount of the urine or in the frequency ?

BLOOD : [Mention it in the H_x of present illness]

Easy fatigability ?
Shortness of breath ?
Awareness of heart beats ' Palpitation ' ?
Bleeding : Red spots in the skin ? , Gum bleeding ? , Nasal bleeding ? , Bruises ? ,
  Rectal bleeding ? , Menstrual disturbances ? , Spontaneous or after trauma ?
H_x of infections ?
Drug H_x : Aspirin , Warfarin , Heparin ?
Family H_x : H_x of blood disorder ?
Glandular enlargement :
Diet : Adequate meat and vegetable consumption ?

PSYCHIATRIC H_x :

PAST MEDICAL H_x :
  Diabetes mellitus , H.T. , Stroke , T.B. , Asthma , … etc.

PAST SURGICAL H_x :
  H_x of previous surgery ? , H_x of trauma , H_x of general anesthesia , H_x of blood transfusion ?

DRUG H_x :
  Drug ? , Dose ? , For how long ? , Why ?
  Allergy to any drug ?

1- MEDICINE — HISTORY TAKING [CASE SHEET]..

FAMILY H_x :

The patient position in the family ?
The age of children , if any ?
State of health ?
Important illness in the family ?
H_x of death in the immediate relatives ? Cause ?
H_x of any hereditary disorder ?

SOCIOECONOMIC H_x :

Started with birth & childhood ..
Marital state (Married , Separated , Divorced or Widow) ?
Living circumstances .. Rural or Urban area ? , Water sanitation ?
Overcrowding in home , pets (animal) in the round ? ,
Education ?
Smoking ? NO. of pack / day , for how many years ? ,
Alcohol .. amount ? type ? duration ?
Any drug addiction ?
Occupation at present time & in the past ? , any associated risk ?
Income & financial state ?
Any H_x of travelling abroad ?

1- MEDICINE — CARDIOVASCULAR system examination..

General Examination:

Hand: clubbing,

splinter hemorrhage,

tobacco stain,

peripheral cyanosis,

xanthoma,

skin temperature,

flapping tremor, capillary refilling

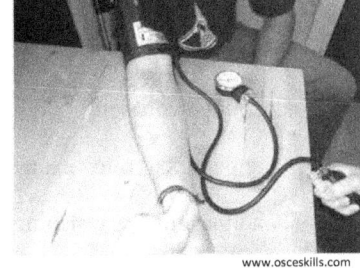
www.osceskills.com

Arm & Forearm: radial pulse, respiratory rate, brachial pulse, B.P.

Head: corneal arcus,

pallor,

xanthelasma,

malar flush,

central cyanosis

Neck: carotid pulse & JVP

Then do complete precordium examination..

Leg: symmetry, swelling, scar, deformity,

hair distribution, skin pigmentation,

temperature, tenderness, edema, sensation,

Trick: Before you touch the patient's leg ask him if he has any pain. During edema examination, you have to see to the face of the patient, if he has any tenderness. And you have to see between the toes for any ischemic changes.

capillary refill time & dorsalis pedis, ant. tibial, post. tibial, popliteal, femoral pulses,

Buerger's test, Trendelenburg test, other tests.. *' for more details you can see vascular examination page 84 '.*

Lung: basal crepitations

Abdomen: ascitis, liver span & tenderness, aortic aneurysm & bruit, sacral edema.

1- MEDICINE   CARDIOVASCULAR system examination..

Precordium examination:

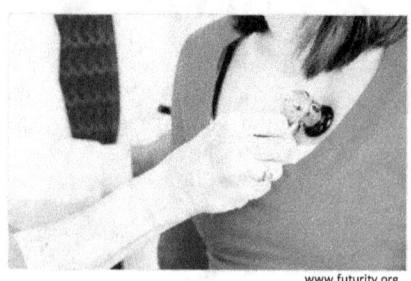

First: greet the patient,

introduce yourself,

take permission for examination,

hand washing & warming,

make sure patient privacy,

good exposure *(explain to the examiner)*

Trick: to see the symmetry, you have to go in front of patient at foot end of the bed..

Inspection: symmetry, skeletal deformity, scar, dilated veins,

pulsation in & outside the precordium. *'APEX BEAT'* is the most important one

Palpation: apex beat *(give its exact site and character)*,

heaving,

thrill *(for murmurs grading)*

Trick: When you feel the apex beat, NEVER remove your fingers then palpate from the sternal angle which is corresponding to the 2nd intercostals space, then see whether it's on the left or right to the mid clavicular line..
Don't forget to palpate the trachea to make sure there is no mediastinal deviation.

Percussion: *not important..*

Auscultation: Mitral (M) *'corresponding to apex beat site'*,

Tricuspid (T),

Pulmonary (P),

Aortic (A) areas..

Trick: You have to palpate the radial pulse to localize the S_1, S_2 and murmurs..

for mitral stenosis *(by the bell and roll the patient to the left side)..*

axillary radiation

aortic regurgitation *(ask the patient to sit and leaning forward and stop respiration for seconds)..*

carotid artery radiation

At the end: cover the patient, thank him..

1- MEDICINE — CARDIOVASCULAR system examination..

Auscultation of precordium:

During the auscultation of precordium, you have to:

identify the first *(S₁)* and second *(S₂)* heart sounds (normal, loud, quiet or splitting),
if there is *S3* or *S4*,
any *added sounds* : friction rub, opening snap (O.S.), ejection click (E.C.),
any *murmur* : timing (systolic, diastolic)
                 character (harsh, rumbling, blowing, ...etc)
                 site of maximum intensity
                 radiation
                 intensity/ grading (1-6)

Trick: You have to palpate the carotid artery or radial pulse (in elderly) to localize the S1, S2 and murmurs..

Radial pulse examination:

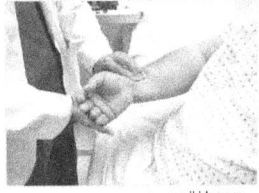

flex the hand slightly,
use 3 finger to palpate the radial artery,
identify *rate, rhythm, volume, character* of the pulse,
collapsing pulse ' *if good volume* ',
radio-femoral delay, then compare the *radial pulse of both hands.*
character of blood vessel wall

JVP examination: ' normal: <4 cm H₂O from sterna angle '

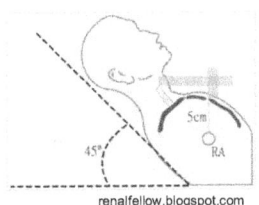

the patient lies at 45°
head to the opposite side, BUT with relaxed neck muscles
inspect from the side

Inspection: rapid inward movement,
         2 peaks per heart beat,
         may vary with patient respiration & position

Palpation: impalpable,
         pulsation decrease by applying pressure at the root of the neck

If *invisible pulse*, then do abdominojugular reflex (5-10 seconds) after asking
         the patient if he has any abdominal pain.

If *very high at 45°*, then ask the patient to sit (90°).

Trick: For previous 3 topics start with greeting the patient, introduce yourself ....etc & end with thank you..

1- MEDICINE   CARDIOVASCULAR system examination..

Heart sounds & murmurs *MADE EASY* **by M.O.M:**

Normal heart sound: **just like** *LUB-DUB*,

When there is S₃: **just like** *LUB-DU-DUB*,

When there is S₄: **just like** *DA-LUB-DUB*

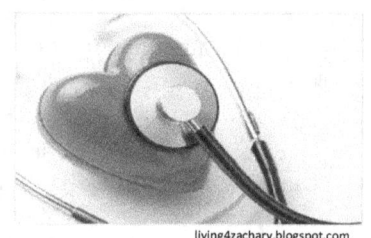

Aortic stenosis: **harsh & rough,**
   Ejection systolic,
   radiated to *neck*

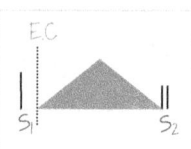

A.S.: Ejection systolic..

Aortic regurgitation: **soft,**
   Early diastolic

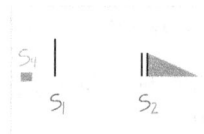

A.R.: Early diastolic..

Mitral stenosis: **Rumbling,**
   Mid-diastolic,
   loud S₁

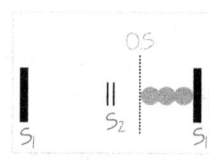

M.S.: Mid-diastolic..

Mitral regurgitation: **soft & blowing,**
   Pansystolic,
   radiated to *axilla*

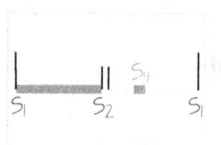

M.R.: Pansystolic..

1- MEDICINE   RESPIRATORY system examination..

General Examination:

General look: wheeze, stridor, type of breathing, cachexia, hoarseness of voice

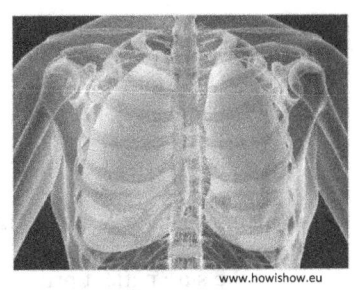

Hand: clubbing,

tobacco stain,

peripheral cyanosis,

flapping tremor, fine tremor ' *drugs side effect e.g. β-agonists used for asthma* ',

capillary refilling

Arm & Forearm: radial pulse, respiratory rate,

skin lesions '*forearm*', B.P.

> Trick: in Respiration you have to identify..
> rate.. ' normal 12-16 cycle/minute ';
> > 20 means tachypnea
> depth.. ' deep or shallow '
> character.. ' acidotic or cheyne-stokes ...etc '
> type.. ' abdominothoracic, thoracic ...etc '

Head: ptosis / Horner's syndrome,

chemosis, conjunctival vessels dilatation,

central cyanosis

Neck: accessory muscles use, JVP, cervical / scalene lymph nodes

---
Then do complete chest examination..

Leg: symmetry, swelling, scar, deformity,

edema ' *bilateral in cor pulmonale & unilateral in D.V.T.* '

Abdomen: liver span ' *hepatomegaly* ', sacral edema.

1- MEDICINE — RESPIRATORY system examination..

Chest examination:

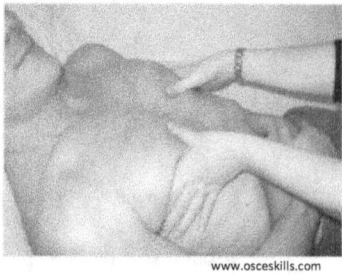

First: greet the patient,

introduce yourself,

take permission for examination,

hand washing & warming,

make sure patient privacy,

good exposure

→ Trick: to see the symmetry, you have to go in front of patient at the foot end of the bed..

Inspection: symmetry, shape, skeletal deformity, scar, rash, pigmentation, dilated veins,

pulsation.. '*APEX BEAT*' is the most important one

Palpation: trachea position and tug

apex beat *(give its exact site and character)*,   ⎤
                                                              ⎬ to identify the position of mediastinum
chest expansion '*with and without tape measure*',

vocal fremitus,

any tenderness, crepitation..

Percussion: don't forget the *apex* of the lung '*above the clavicle*',

clavicle '*directly on the bone*',

chest wall '*upper, middle, base, lateral..*'

Auscultation: apex of the lung then the chest wall '*upper, middle, base, lateral..*'

identify.. breath sounds,

any added sounds (*rhonchi, crepitation, rub*),

vocal resonant,

whispering pectoriloquy..

At the end: cover the patient, thank him..

1- MEDICINE — RESPIRATORY system examination..

DON'T FORGET *the examination of the chest from the* BACK..

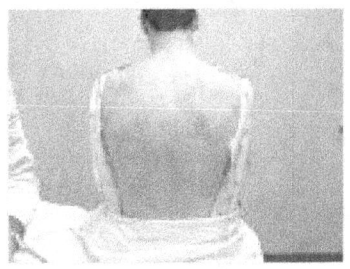

Chest examination from the back:

It is the same as the chest examination ' *mentioned in the previous page* ', BUT with *some exceptions* :

Ask the patient to cross his hands and put them over his shoulders..

- Inspection: symmetry, shape, skeletal deformity, scar *only*
- Palpation: chest expansion, vocal fremitus *only*
- Percussion: *apex* & chest wall ' *upper, middle, base, lateral..* '

Trick: at the level of right 5th thoracic rib the dullness is either pathological or normal liver dullness.. so, ask the patient to take deep breath, if the dullness disappear so it is liver dullness otherwise it is underlying lesion. This is called ' *tidal percussion* '.

otherTrick: Technique for percussion..
The percussing finger (plexor) should be sharply struck against the distal interphalangeal joint of the middle finger of the opposite hand (pleximeter). The motion should be generated at the *wrist* rather than with the whole arm, then *remove the plexor* (don't keep it in touch with the pleximeter), otherwise all your percussion will be dull.

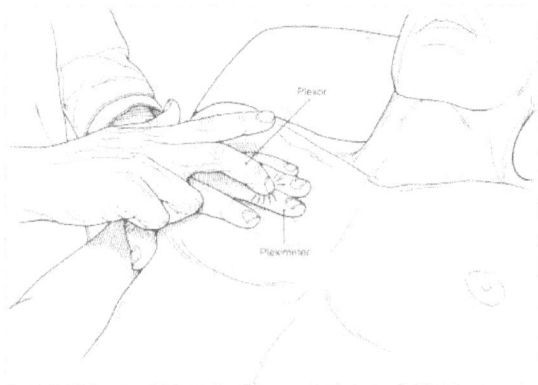

1- MEDICINE — GASTROINTESTINAL system examination..

General Examination:

General look: nutritional state

Hand: clubbing,

koilonychia, leuconychia,

palmar creases *'pallor'*, palmar erythema,

Dupuytren's contracture,

flapping tremor

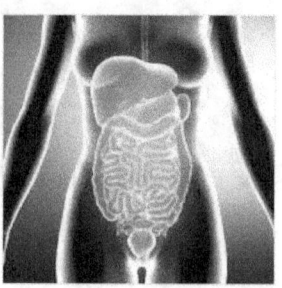

Arm & Forearm: radial pulse, respiratory rate, B.P.

Head: pallor, jaundice, *Kayser-Fleischer ring*,

parotid swelling,

angular stomatitis, glossitis, tongue, odor of the mouth

Neck: left supraclvicular lymph node

Chest: spider naevi, gynecomastia

Then do complete abdominal examination..

Leg: edema, pyoderma gangrenosum

Mention at the end: the inguinal region *(hernial orifices, lymph nodes)*,

back examination,

per-rectum examination

left supraclavicular lymph node

1- MEDICINE   GASTROINTESTINAL system examination..

Abdomen examination:

First: greet the patient,

introduce yourself,

take permission for examination,

hand washing & warming,

make sure patient privacy,

good exposure *' from above the nipple to the mid-thigh ', may not done due to social embarrassment..*

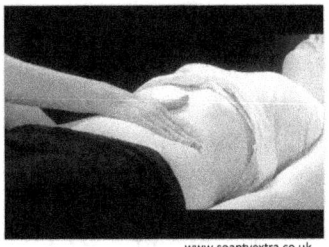

www.soaptvextra.co.uk

Inspection: *symmetry*, shape of the abdomen & umbilicus, any distension,

movement with respiration, scar, stria, rash, pigmentation, dilated veins,

hair distribution, gynecomastia,

peristaltic wave, pulsation,

hernia *(ask the patient to cough)..*

→ Trick: to see the symmetry, you have to go in front of patient at the bed end..

Palpation: *' rub your hands, knee sitting, ask if he has any pain.., see to the face of the patient & you can ask him to flex his knee slightly to relax abdominal muscles '..*

superficial: tenderness & rebound tenderness, mass, and rigidity

deep: liver, spleen *' two methods '*, kidneys, urinary bladder,

aorta, lymph nodes, *femoral vessels,* anterior abdominal wall edema

→ Trick: may need dipping method in huge ascitis..

Percussion: liver span *(normally 10±2)*, spleen, shifting dullness and transmitted thrill, urinary bladder, kidneys *' from the back.. '* ↘

Trick: after you ask the patient to roll to his side, you have to wait for about 30 seconds..

Auscultation: bowel sounds, renal artery and aorta bruit, liver & spleen friction sounds

At the end: cover the patient, thank him..

1- MEDICINE — GASTROINTESTINAL system examination..

Now, the question is ' *HOW TO DIFFERENTIATE BETWEEN the enlargement of the SPLEEN from the LEFT KIDNEY ??* '

The answer is ' *by palpation & percussion..* ' & the differences are as the following :

Enlarged **SPLEEN**	Enlarged **LEFT KIDNEY**
1- *Sharp* edge	1- **Round** edge
2- *Notch* is present in its superomedial edge	2- **Not** present
3- Enlarges *downward & medially*	3- **Downward only**
4- Bimanually *impalpable*	4- Bimanually **palpable**
5- You *can't get above it*	5- **Can get above** it (between the palpable mass and the costal margin)
6- *Dull* note on percussion	6- **Resonant** on percussion

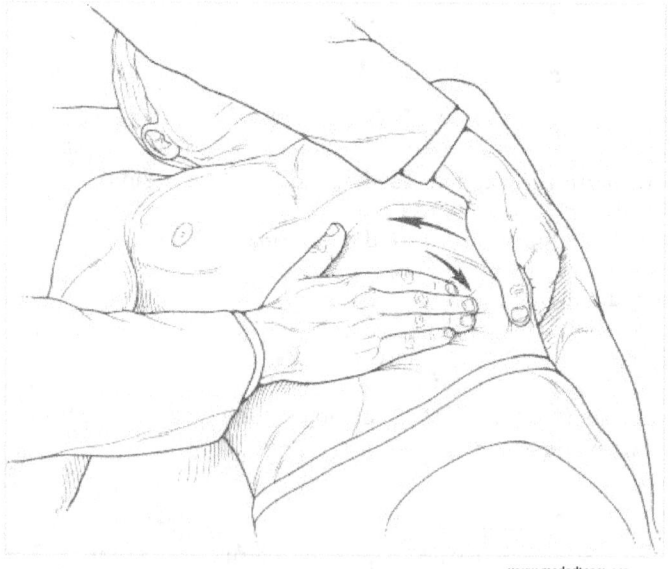

www.medadteam.org

1- MEDICINE — GENERAL EXAMINATION..

General examination:

First: greet the patient,

introduce yourself,

take permission for examination,

hand washing & warming,

make sure patient privacy,

good exposure *' when needed..'*

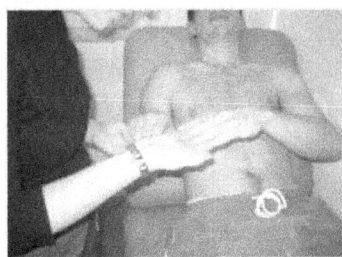

General look: *' for example '*, a middle age ♀, lying flat in the bed,

she look well, comfortable, conscious, alert, oriented *(for place, person and time)*,

not dyspneic, no wheeze, no stridor with one pillow under her head,

no specific complexion *' like earthy color for example '*,

with green i.v. cannula in her right hand, no i.v. fluid, no O_2 bottle ....etc

good nutritional state

Head: hair, eye brow, puffiness around the eye,

eye → corneal arcus, pallor, jaundice, ptosis, lid retraction, exophthalmos, squint, hemorrhage

xanthelasma, malar flush or rash, parotid swelling,

ear

mouth → angular stomatitis, pallor,

tongue ' cyanosis, dry or wet, glossitis, thrush ',

gums ' hypertrophied, bleeding ',

teeth ' dental caries ',

any ulcer or pigmentations *(use torch light)*

Neck: lymph nodes, J.V.P., carotid artery, thyroid, use of accessory respiratory muscles

1- MEDICINE — GENERAL EXAMINATION..

Hand: symmetry, any deformity, muscle wasting, scar,

swelling, redness,

nail ' *clubbing, cyanosis*, splinter hemorrhage,

koilonychia, leuconychia, half and half nail ',

xanthoma,

pallor, palmar erythema, dupuytren contracture,

hot or cold, wet or dry,

fine & flapping tremor,

capillary refilling

Schamroth's window test - www.osceskills.com
when there is clubbing.. the diamond space will loss..

Trick: finger's clubbing stages:
stage.. 1 - Fluctuation and softening of the nail bed
2- Loss of the normal <165° angle
3- Increased convexity of the nail fold
4- Thickening of the whole distal finger (drumstick)
5- Shiny aspect and striation of the nail and skin

Arm & forearm: any skin lesion, radial pulse & respiratory rate, B.P., temperature

brachial artery, epitrochlear lymph nodes,

Leg: symmetry, hair distribution, ulcer, skin lesion, *swelling, edema, D.V.T signs*,

capillary refilling time & dorsalis pedis, ant. tibial, post. tibial, popliteal, femoral pulses,

Trick: Before you touch the patient's leg ask him if he has any pain. During edema examination, you have to see to the face of the patient, if he has any tenderness. And you have to see between the toes for any ischemic changes.

chest: spider naevi, gynecomastia, deformity, skin lesion & *axillary lymph nodes*.

Abdomen: distension, scar, stria, dilated veins, para-aortic lymph nodes, femoral artery,

inguinal lymph nodes, popliteal lymph nodes,

back: sacral edema, others...

Trick: *NEVER* mention the steps in GREY color in the exam.

At the end: cover the patient, thank him..

★★ *For proper* **Hand & Wrist EXAMINATION***, you can see page 120 ..*

1- MEDICINE — NERVOUS system examination..

General examination:

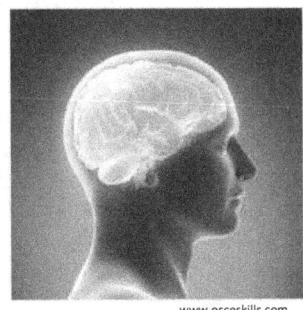

First: greet the patient,

introduce yourself,

take permission for examination,

hand washing & warming,

make sure patient privacy,

good exposure *' when needed..'*

Consciousness: level *' full conscious, drowsy, stupor or comatose '*,

content *' full conscious, confuse, delirious (confused + agitated), comatose '*

Mental state: memory *' immediate, short & long term '*,

reasoning & judgment *' similarity & dissimilarity, solving problems,*

giving explanation ',

attention & concentration

speech: comprehension,

fluency,

reading,

writing,

repetition,

naming,

Trick: you can do this by these orders in sequence..:
stand behind the patient & ask him to raise his right arm..
talk to me about your problem..
write to him ' close your eyes..'
ask him to write about his problem..
repeat this sentence ' we are at Baghdad hospital. '
show him a pen & ask him ' what is this ? '

and during the examination you have to..

observe the *volume, rhythm & clarity* of speech,

ask him to count from 1 to 30 and see if she get tired,

say ahhhh, cough, say ' SALSABEEL or COSTANTINYA ' in Arabic.

1- MEDICINE — NERVOUS system examination..

Stance & gait: **ask him to stand open then closed their eyes**
' stand behind the patient to pevent him from falling on the ground.. ',

ask him to walk *' observe if he need any assistance, arm swing, steadiness, limping ',*

tandem gait, tip toe walking

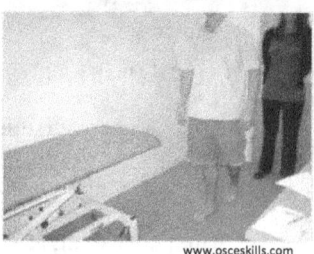

www.osceskills.com

Meningeal signs: *you have to ask the patient if he has any neck pain or trauma,*

exposure *' his legs.. ',*

neck stiffness: **move the head from one side to other,**

neck flexion *' till the chin touch the chest ',*

see if there is reflex knee flexion *(BRUDZINSKI'S sign)*

Kernig's sign: **flex the knee & hip joints,**

then do knee extension and see if there is any resistance to knee extension

↓

Trick: here, you have to put your hand on the Hamstrings muscle..

KERNIG'S SIGN	BRUDZINSKI'S NECK SIGN
Elicitation: Flexing the patient's hip 90 degrees then extending the patient's knee causes pain.	**Elicitation:** Flexing the patient's neck causes flexion of the patient's hips and knees.

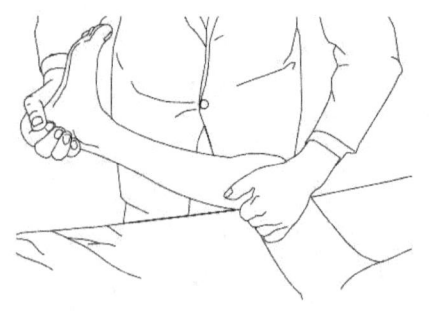

Saberi & Syed Meningeal Signs

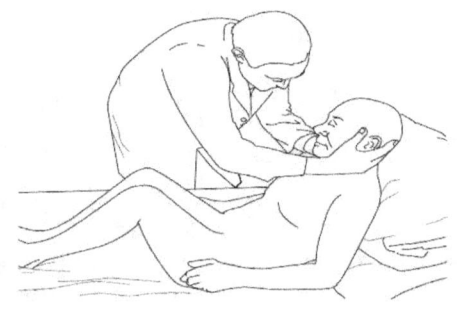

Saberi & Syed Meningeal Signs

At the end: **cover the patient, thank him..**

1- MEDICINE — NERVOUS system examination..

Cranial nerves:

1st – Olfactory n.: patent airway ' by inspection ',

3 tubes with different familiar odor

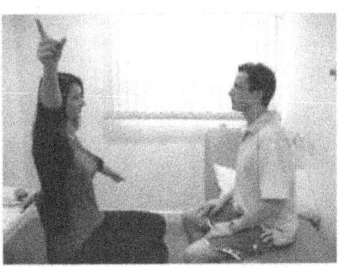

2nd – Optic n.: visual acuity *' for distant & near vision '*,

visual field *'by confrontation test & red pin '*,

papillary reflexes ' **light** & *accommodation* ',

color vision, fundoscopy

3rd, 4th, 6th – Oculomotor, Trochlear, Abducent nn.:

inspect for *ptosis, proptosis & squint*,

Trick: if present, ask the patient to cover one eye then the other.. when the affected eye is covered, the peripheral (false) image will disappear.

movement of the eye ' any squint, nystagmus, diplopia during examination ',

reflexes ' *papillary (direct & indirect) and accommodation* '

5th – Trigeminal n.: *motor..*

inspect for muscles wasting ' *masseter, temporalis, pterygoid* ',

palpate the bulk of the masseter & temporalis,

open the jaw against resistance,

sensory..

light touch & superficial pain ' *for maxillary, mandibular, ophthalmic branches* ',

anterior 2/3 of the tongue (but not taste),

reflexes..

corneal reflex,

jaw jerk

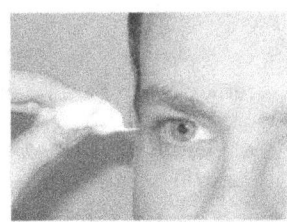

1- MEDICINE — NERVOUS system examination..

7th – Facial n.: asymmetry, involuntary movement, blinking of the eye,

4 orders: ' MOST COMMON ORDERS in nervous system.. '

raise your eyebrows.. *' see the asymmetry of the forehead creases ',*

show me your teeth.. *' see mouth deviation ',*

close your eyes.. *' try to open it ',* → Trick: only lower part affected = U.M.N.L
Upper & lower part affected = L.M.N.L

puff out your cheeks *' against resistant ',*

anterior 2/3 of the tongue *' taste sensation ',*

satpedius muscle *' hyperacusis ',*

corneal reflex *' because the facial is efferent '*

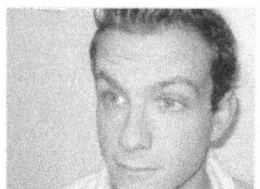 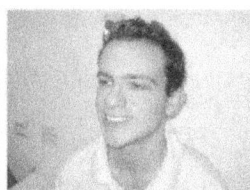 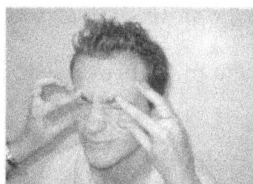 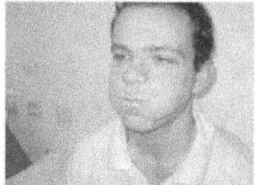

www.osceskills.com

8th – Vestibulocochlear n.: whisper, Rinne's test & Weber's test..

9th – Glossopharyngeal n.: sensation & taste in the posterior 1/3 of the tongue, gag reflex

10th – Vagus n.: say Ahhhhh, ask him to cough *' bovine cough ',* dysphonea

→ Trick: Examine the 9th & 10th together..:
speech,
drink,
say Ahhhhh, please cough,
gag reflex, posterior pharyngeal wall sensation,
sensation in the posterior 1/3 of the tongue..

11th – Accessory n.: **sternocleidomastoid..** *inspection, palpation,* turn their head against resistance..

trapezius.. *inspection, palpation,* ask the patient to shrug their shoulders

1- MEDICINE — NERVOUS system examination..

12th – Hypoglossal n.: open your mouth *' any wasting, fasciculation, involuntary movement '*,

protrude the tongue *' deviation or involuntary movement '*,

move it from one side to other,

power of the tongue,

speech *' say yellow lorry.. '*

DON'T FORGET.. AS ANY EXAMINATION:

First: greet the patient,

introduce yourself,

take permission for examination,

hand washing,

make sure patient privacy,

good exposure *' when needed.. '*

Then do complete Cranial nerve examination..

At the end: cover the patient, thank him..

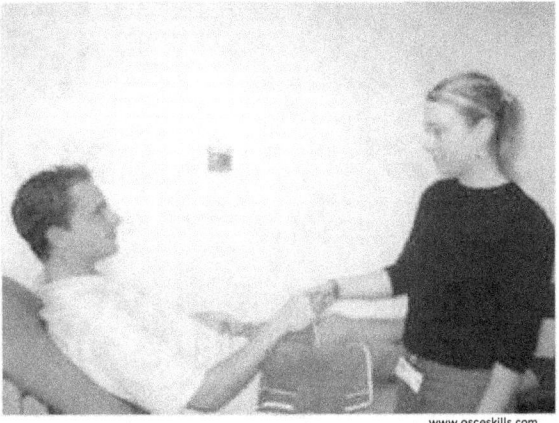

1- MEDICINE — NERVOUS system examination..

Upper limb *motor* examination:

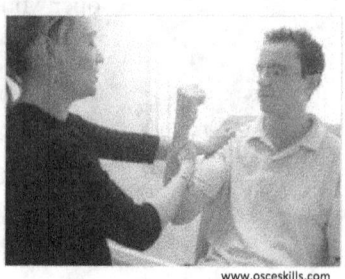

First: greet the patient,
introduce yourself,
take permission for examination,
hand washing,
make sure patient privacy,
good exposure *' when needed..'*

Inspection & Palpation: symmetry, deformity, posture,
any wasting,
involuntary movement *'fasciculation, tremor, myoclonic jerk, other '*

Trick: spontaneous or induced by taping on the muscles..

Tone: shoulder, elbow, wrist, fingers..

Reflexes: biceps C_5-C_6,
triceps C_6-C_7,
supinator C_5-C_6,   — If -ve, do reinforcement..

finger jerk C_8-T_1,
hoffman's sign $C_{7,8}$-T_1

Trick: Grades of reflexes..
clonus ++++
brisk +++
normal ++
decrease +
with reinforcement ±
absent -

Power: shoulder *' abduction & adduction '*,
elbow *' flexion & extension '*,
wrist *' flexion & extension '*,
fingers *' abduction & adduction, flexion & extension then the thumb..'*

Function: like dressing apraxia, construction apraxia, dyspraxia..

At the end: cover the patient, thank him..

1- MEDICINE — NERVOUS system examination..

Lower limb *motor* examination:

First: greet the patient,

introduce yourself,

take permission for examination,

hand washing,

make sure patient privacy,

good exposure *'when needed..'*

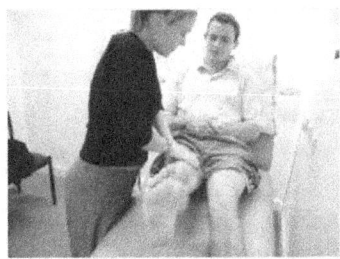

Inspection & Palpation: symmetry, deformity, posture,

any wasting,

involuntary movement *'fasciculation, tremor, myoclonic jerk, other'*

Trick: spontaneous or induced by taping on the muscles..

Tone: roll the leg on the bed to see if it moves easily,

pull up on the knee to check its tone,

hip, knee, ankle, toes

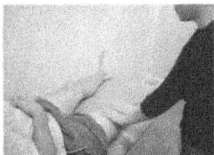 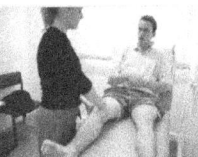

rolling of the leg & pulling up of the knee - www.osceskills.com

Reflexes: knee L₃-L₄,
ankle S₁-S₂,

If –ve, do reinforcement..

planter S₁-S₂

Trick: Grades of reflexes..
clonus ++++
brisk +++
normal ++
decrease +
with reinforcement ±
absent -

Clonus: patellar, ankle

Power: hip *'flexion & extension, abduction & adduction'*,
knee *'flexion & extension'*,
ankle *'dorsiflexion & plantarflexion'*,
toes *'dorsiflexion & plantarflexion'*,

At the end: cover the patient, thank him..

1- MEDICINE   NERVOUS system examination..

Coordination:

First: greet the patient,

introduce yourself,

take permission for examination,

hand washing,

make sure patient privacy,

good exposure ' when needed..'

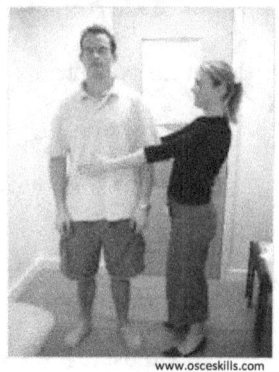

Specific: *upper limb..* finger nose test, rapid alternating movement, rebound phenomena,

lower limb.. heel-shin test, heel toe (tandem) gait, Romberg's test..

non-specific: speech ability, nystagmus,

At the end: cover the patient, thank him..

Sensory examination:

Light touch: by cotton,

Superficial & deep pain: by pinprick,

Temperature:

Vibration:

Joint position sensation: (proprioception),

2 points discrimination:

Stereognosis: for familial objects

Graphesthesia:

Finger touch:

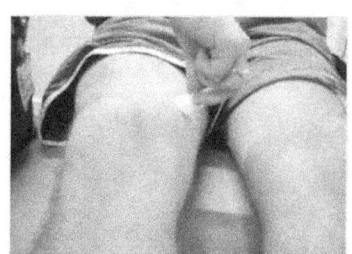

Trick: there are 2 method for touch and pain sensation examination.. either to dermatome distribution or sensory level.

1- MEDICINE — NERVOUS system examination..

Hand nerve supply examination:

General: wasting,

Motor: *median n...* thumb abduction & apposition,

  ulnar n... adduction of little finger, abduction of index, thumb adduction,

  radial n... finger extension, wrist extension, thumb extension,

Sensory: *median n...* palmar surface of the index,

  ulnar n.. medial surface of the palm,

  radial n... dorsum of the hand just below the cleft between the thumb & index..

Trick: Technique of tendon reflex examination..
  make sure the limb is relaxed,
  palpate the tendon,
  put the hammer on the tendon ' in touch with it ',
  then gentle percussion..
  if –ve, then do reinforcement..

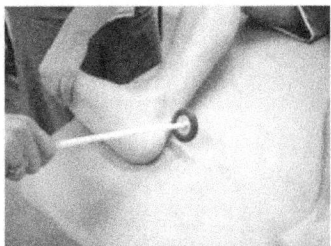

Trick: Grades of the power..
  grade 0 - *no movement,*
  grade 1 - *muscle contraction* only (no joint movement),
  grade 2 - joint move only *with gravity,*
  grade 3 - move against gravity,
  grade 4 - against gravity but *with some degree of weakness against resistance,*
  grade 5 – NORMAL

So, start by asking the patient to raise his limbs.. if he can do it against gravity, so..the grade roughly is more than 3.

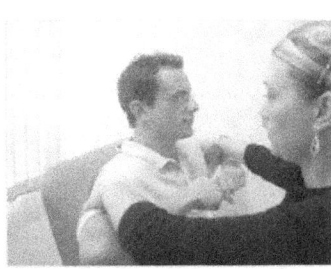

CHAPTER 2

ECG
by Dr. M.O.M

Contents:

INTRODUCTION	38
WAVES & INTERVALS	42
CARDIAC AXIS	46
HYPERTROPHY	48
ISCHEMIC HEART DISEASE	49
HEART BLOCK	51
DYSARRHYTHMIA	53
HYPERKALEMIA & HYPOKALEMIA	56
PERICARDITIS VS. INFARCTION	57
HOW TO READ & REPORT THE ECG	58
OTHER TOPICS	59

2- ECG by M.O.M — INTRODUCTION..

ECG by M.O.M – INTRODUCTION

In this chapter, I would like to explain some practical points in the *basics of the ECG interpretation*.. and answer the two important questions..
' *HOW TO READ THE ECG ?* ' &
' *HOW TO REPORT THE ECG ?* '..

So, by the end of this chapter you should have a systematic approach to interpreting the ECG and be able to identify the common ECG abnormalities.

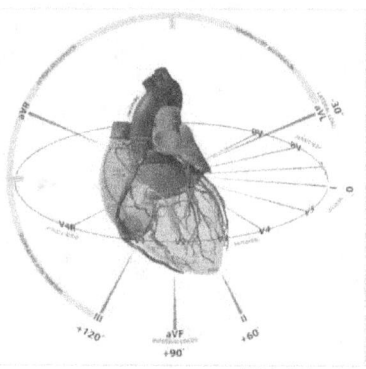

www.lifeinthefastlane.com

The 12 lead ECG:

The 12 lead ECG is made up of the three standard limb leads (I, II and III), the augmented limb leads (aVR, aVL and aVF) and the six precordial leads (V1, V2, V3, V4, V5 and V6).

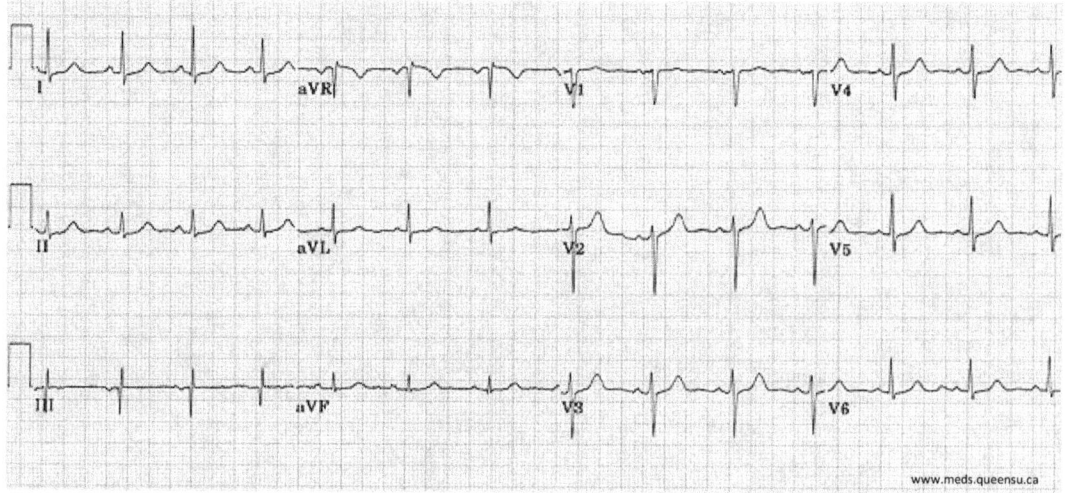

A normal ECG is illustrated above. Note that the heart is beating in a regular sinus rhythm between 60 - 100 beats per minute (specifically 82 bpm). All the important intervals on this recording are within normal ranges.

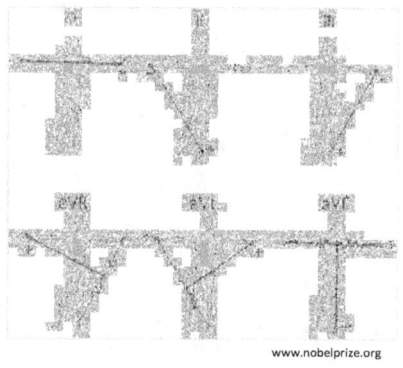

www.nobelprize.org

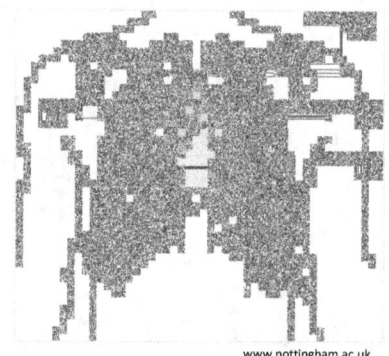

www.nottingham.ac.uk

2- ECG by M.O.M — INTRODUCTION..

Trick: ' NEVER FORGET THIS TOPIC.. '

Localization of the abnormality

the directions from which the various leads look at the heart:

V1-V4   anteroseptal wall

V5-V6   lateral wall

    V1-V2   septal wall
    V3-V4   anterior wall
    V5-V6   lateral wall

II, III, aVF   inferior wall

I, aVL   lateral wall

V1-V2   **posterior wall** *(reciprocal)*

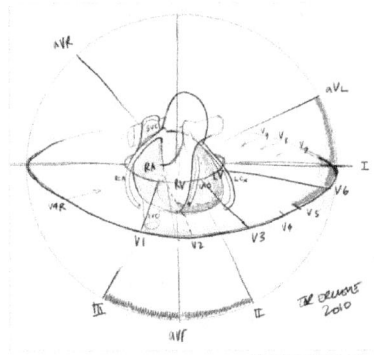

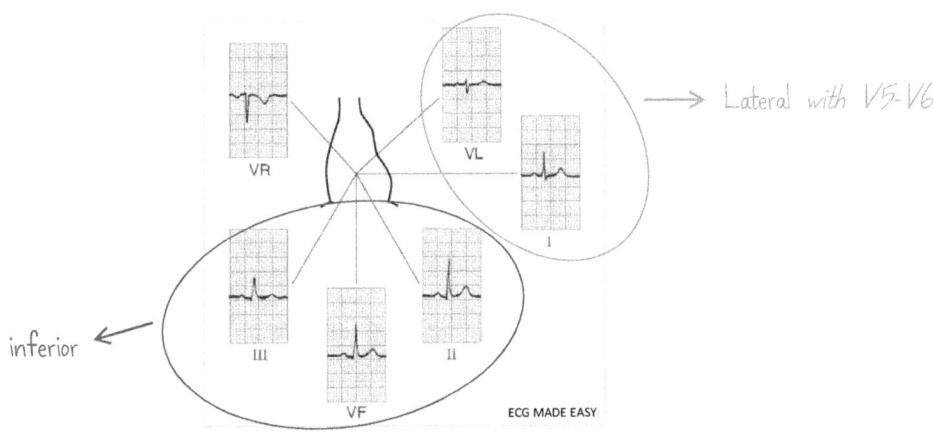

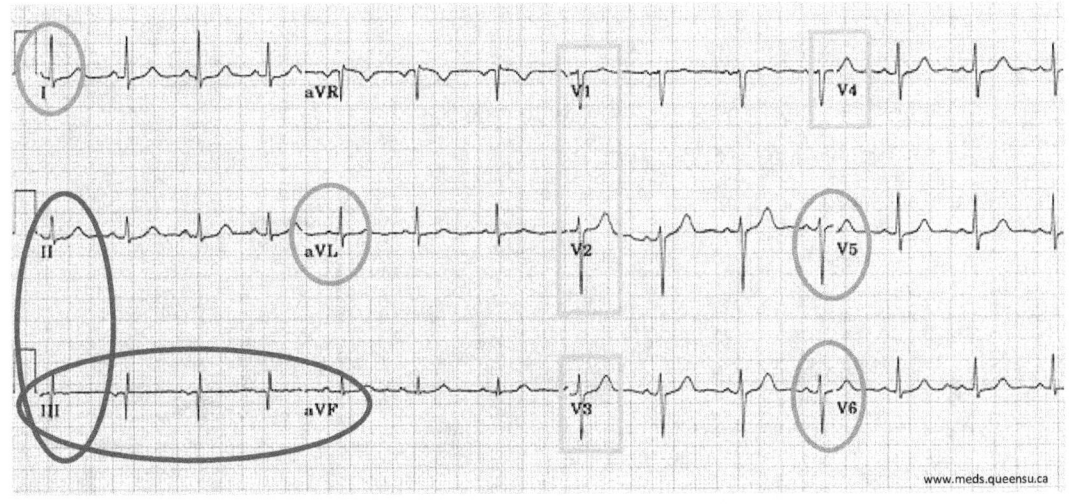

2- ECG by M.O.M — INTRODUCTION..

ECG thermal paper:

the ECG paper consists from large (☐) & small (□) squares.. the relationship between the squares on ECG paper, time & voltage is explained in the figure below:

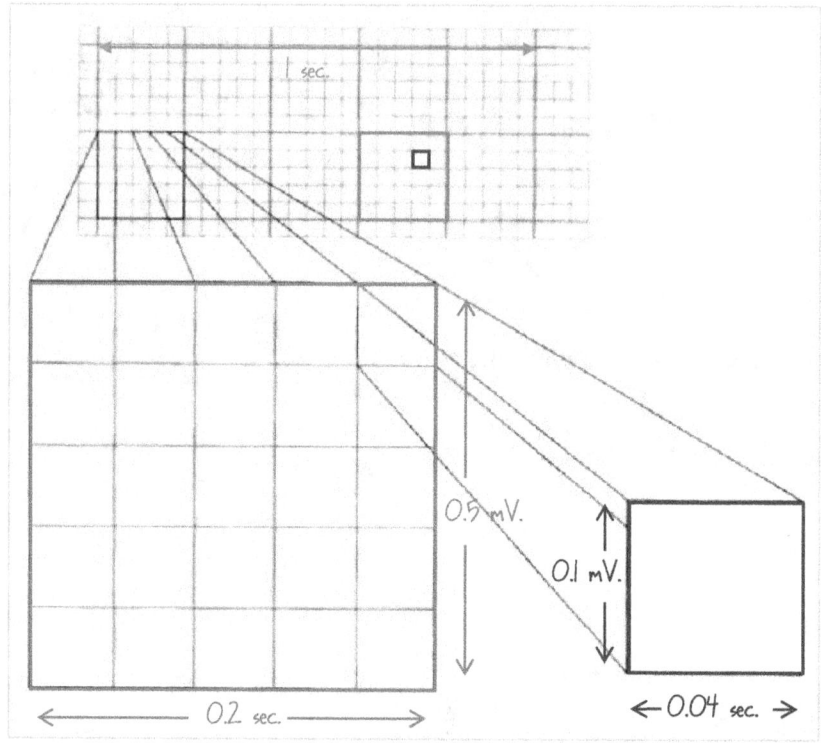

www.scribd.com – understanding ECG

Calibration & Speed:

it is important to make sure normal calibration & speed in every ECG..

normal calibration = 1mV. = 1cm. &

normal speed = 25 mm./sec..

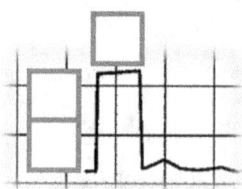

Trick: so, 2 large squares X 1 large square is a must..

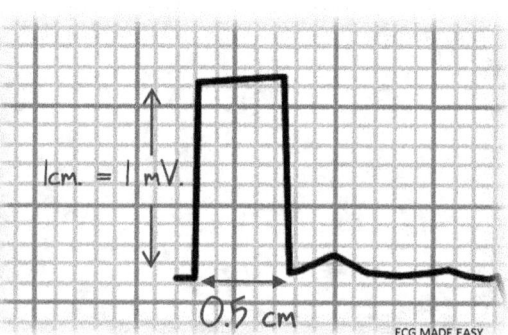

ECG MADE EASY

Heart rate:

The *ideal way* to calculate the heart rate is by count the no. of small or *large* squares between the 2 consecutive R waves, then calculate the heart rate by one of these equations:

Heart rate = 1500 / no. of R-R □   or   Heart rate = 300 / no. of R-R □

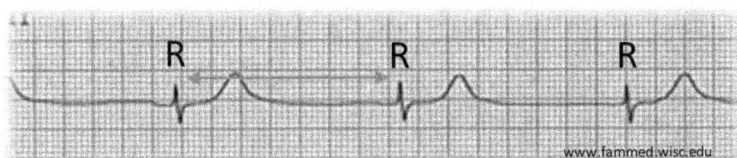

Count number of large boxes between first and second R waves=7.5.. 300/7.5 large boxes = rate 40

★★ You can use S wave as well..

Trick: The practical way to calculate the rate is depend on the no. of large squares between 2 consecutive R waves and as the following..

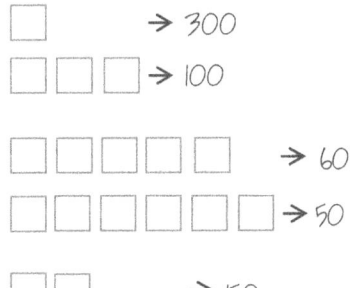

□ → 300
□□□ → 100
□□□□□ → 60
□□□□□□ → 50
□□ → 150
□□□□ → 75

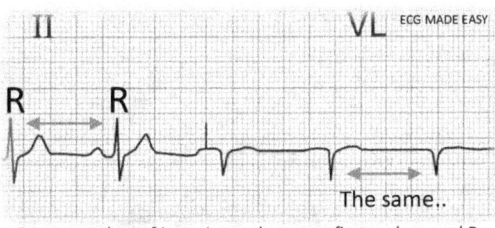

Count number of large boxes between first and second R waves = 4.. So, the heart rate = 75

if you have an *irregular rhythm* (like atrial fibrillation).. so, when you want to know an average rate, you can use the six-second method:

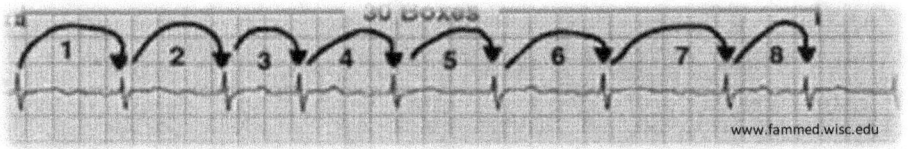

Count 30 large boxes, starting from the first R wave. There are 8 R-R intervals within 30 boxes. Multiply 8 x 10 = Rate 80.

2- ECG by M.O.M — WAVES & INTERVALS..

Waves & intervals:

The picture of an ECG consists of several waves, complexes, intervals & segments..
So, I would like to explain each of these components individually..
BUT, first you have to know some of their definitions and general idea to be oriented... :

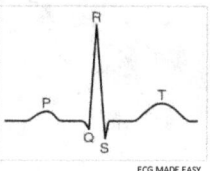
ECG MADE EASY

Waves & complexes:

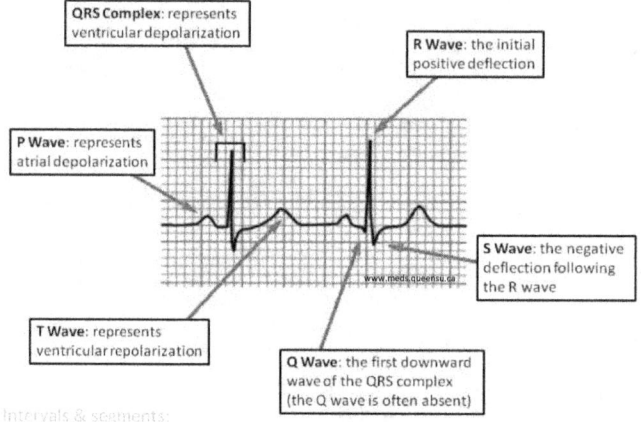

- **QRS Complex**: represents ventricular depolarization
- **R Wave**: the initial positive deflection
- **P Wave**: represents atrial depolarization
- **S Wave**: the negative deflection following the R wave
- **T Wave**: represents ventricular repolarization
- **Q Wave**: the first downward wave of the QRS complex (the Q wave is often absent)

Intervals & segments:

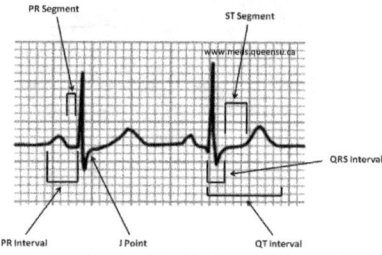

PR Interval:	From the start of the P wave to the start of the QRS complex
PR Segment:	From the end of the P wave to the start of the QRS complex
J Point:	The junction between the QRS complex and the ST segment
QT Interval:	From the start of the QRS complex to the end of the T wave
QRS Interval:	From the start to the end of the QRS complex
ST Segment:	From the end of the QRS complex (J point) to the start of the T wave

2- ECG by M.O.M — WAVES & INTERVALS..

Trick: no. of □ × 0.04 = time in seconds..

P wave:

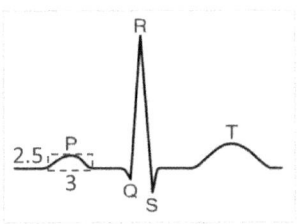

normally: 3□ × 2.5□

+ve except in (aVR −ve)

In **lead I** : almost always +ve..
If −ve → either *wrong connection* or *dextrocardi*

In left atrium enlargement: *bifid P* wave in leads I, aVL, may be II
biphasic in V_1

In right atrium enlargement: *tented P wave* in leads II, III, aVF & V_1

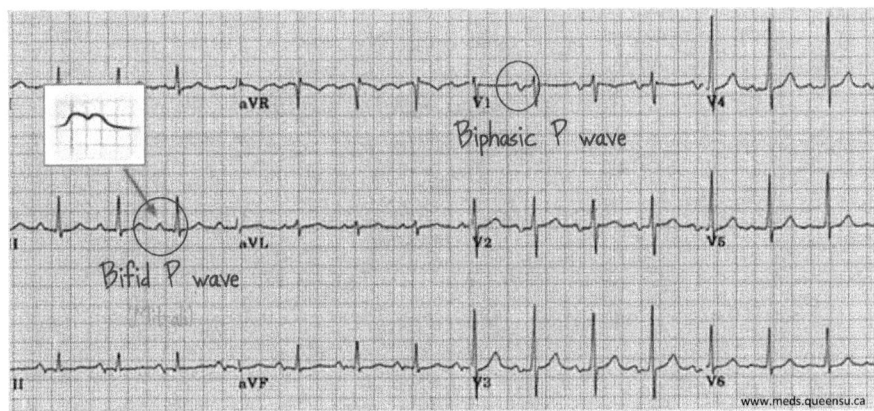

Left atrial enlargement: the P wave in lead II is bifid & the P wave in lead V_1 is biphasic (has terminal negative deflection)..

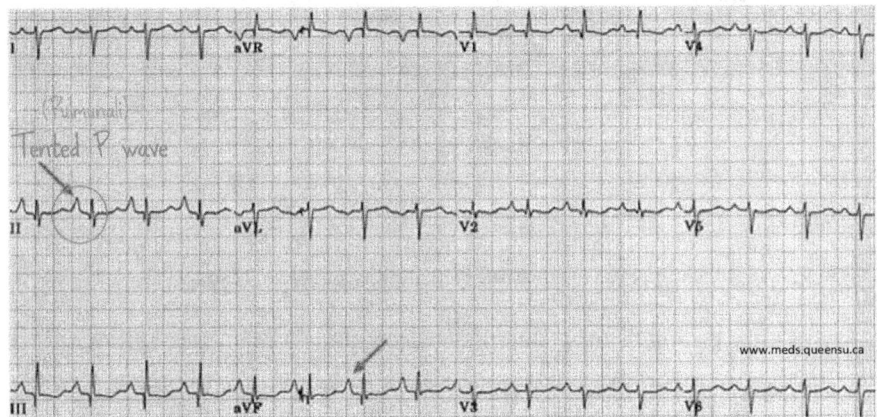

Right atrial enlargement: the P wave in lead II is tented (has amplitude of 4 small squares)..

2- ECG by M.O.M — WAVES & INTERVALS..

P-R interval:

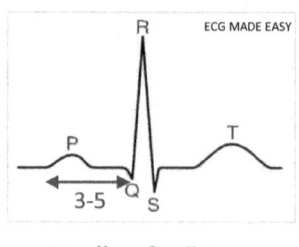

normally = 3 – 5 □

QRS complex:

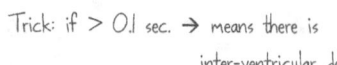

Trick: if > 0.1 sec. → means there is inter-ventricular delay..

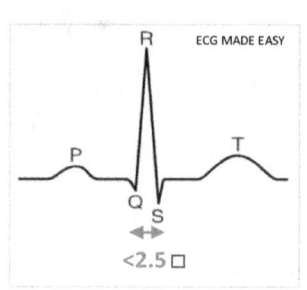

<2.5 □

normally = (0.06-0.1 sec.)

Q wave:

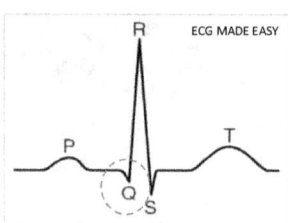

normally in aVR..

normal *septal Q* wave → **< 25%** of R wave
  < □ (0.04 sec.)

pathological Q wave → **> 25%** of R wave or
  > □ (0.04 sec.)

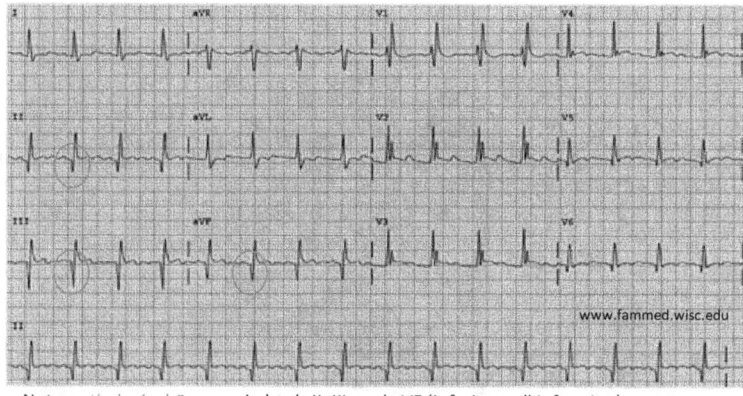

Note *pathological Q waves* in leads II, III, and aVF (inferior wall infarction)..

ST segment:

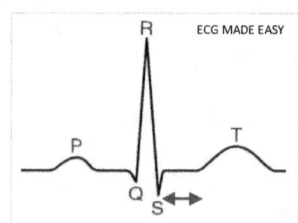

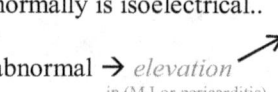

normally is isoelectrical..

abnormal → *elevation*
  in (M.I or pericarditis)

or *depression* →
  in (ischemia, electrolyte disturbances, ventricular hypertrophy)

T wave:

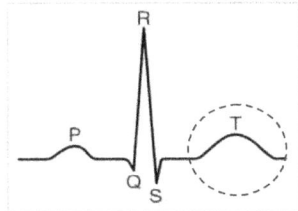

normally: +ve in leads I, II, V$_{3-6}$

inverted in aVR

variable in the other leads

normal height → *5 mm.* in *limb* leads (one ☐)

10 mm. in *chest leads* (two ☐)

more than this range it is consider as a *tall, tented T wave*.. like in: M.I, ↑K⁺, C.V.A..

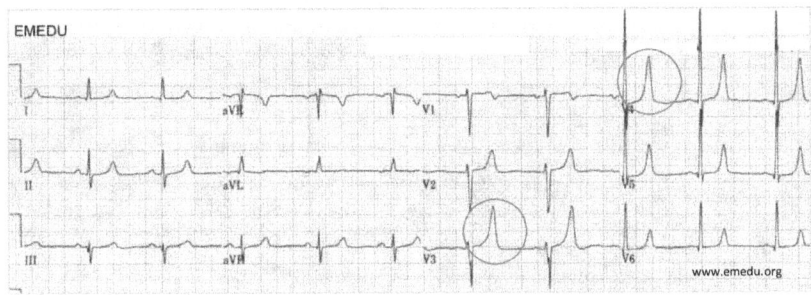

Hyperkalemia: Note the *tall, tented T waves*..

QT interval:

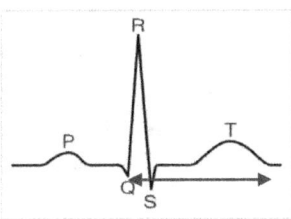

normally : 8 – 11.5 ☐ (0.32 – 0.46 sec.)
prolonged in → heart failure, ↓Ca^{+2}, drugs

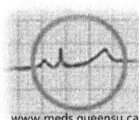

U wave:

is a small (0.5 mm) deflection *immediately following the T wave*, usually in the same direction as the T wave, may be normal in ECG, especially in V$_3$..

prominant in ↓K⁺ & opposite to T wave in myocardial ischemia..

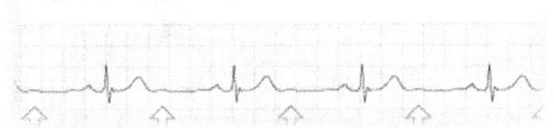

U wave.. U wave.. U wave.. U wave..

2- ECG by M.O.M — THE CARDIAC AXIS..

Calculation of the electrical axis:

The mean QRS axis refers to the average orientation of the heart's electrical activity. In most cases, an approximation of the axis will be sufficient for the ECG interpretation. There are many different approaches to axis determination, but this discussion will be limited to two approaches only ' *the practical & ideal approaches* '..

Trick:

The practical approaches: is depends on the QRS deflection in the leasds I, II, III..

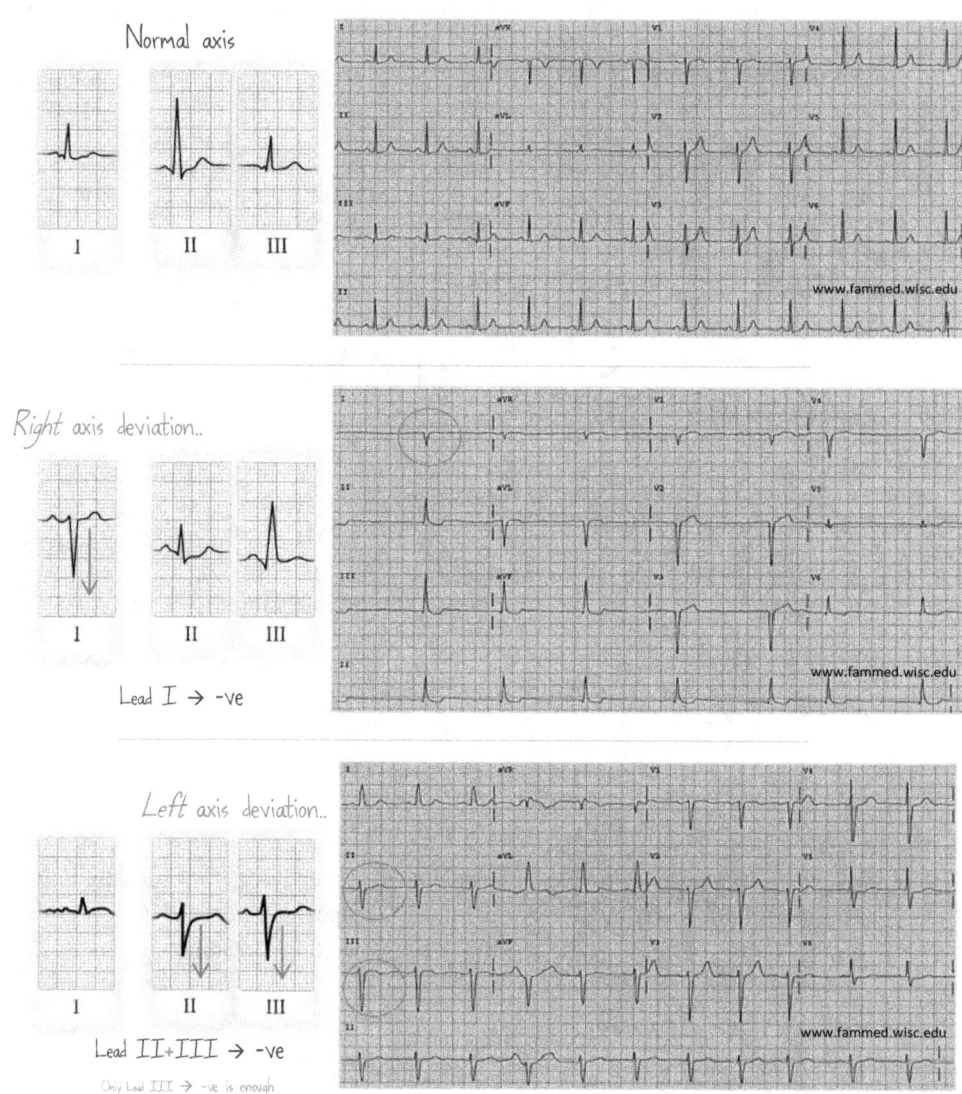

Normal axis
I   II   III

Right axis deviation..
I   II   III
Lead I → -ve

Left axis deviation..
I   II   III
Lead II+III → -ve
Only Lead III → -ve is enough

M.O.M's OSCEs : The 1st Book from M.A.S and M.O.M series..

The ideal approach:

The mean QRS axis is oriented towards the lead with the greatest net QRS deflection. To calculate the net QRS deflection, add up the number of small squares that correspond to the height of the R wave (positive deflection), and subtract the number of small squares that correspond to the height of the Q and S waves (negative deflection).

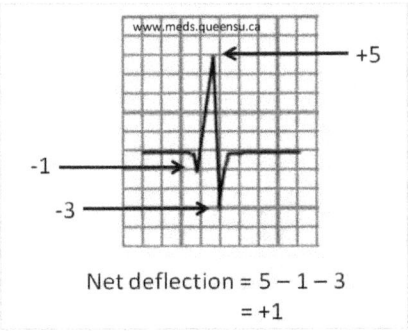

Net deflection = 5 − 1 − 3
= +1

Approximate the net QRS deflection for leads I and aVF. Remember that the mean QRS axis will be oriented towards the lead with the greatest positive net QRS deflection. If the net deflection is positive for both, the axis lies between leads I and aVF (0-90°) and is therefore normal.

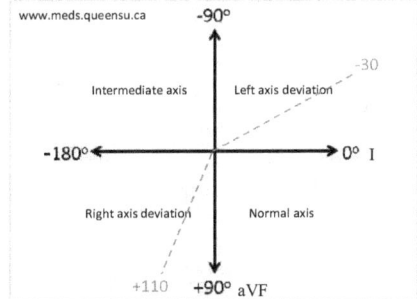

You have to remember this image to use this approach..

For example..

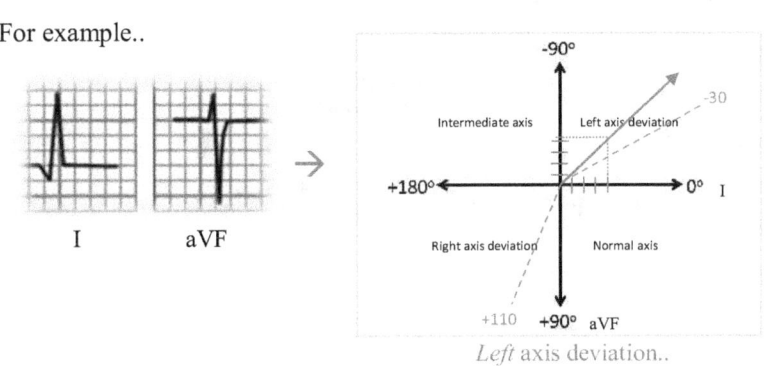

Left axis deviation..

2- ECG by M.O.M — HYPERTROPHY

Ventricular hypertrophy:

Left ventricular hypertrophy (L.V.H.):

If.. The S wave in V_1
+
The R wave in $V_{5\ or\ 6}$

$> 35\ □\ →\ L.V.H.$

Note: if the L.V.H. is *sever*, you will see ST depression and T wave inversion in the lateral leads I, aVL & V_{5-6}..

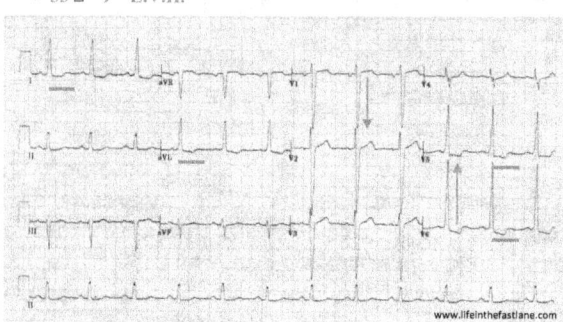

Left ventricular hypertrophy (L.V.H.)..

Right ventricular hypertrophy (R.V.H.):

If.. The $R ≥ S$ wave in V_1
The $S ≥ R$ wave in V_6

Note: if the R.V.H. is *sever*, you will see ST depression &T wave inversion in the V_{2-3} due to hypertrophy (not M.I.)..

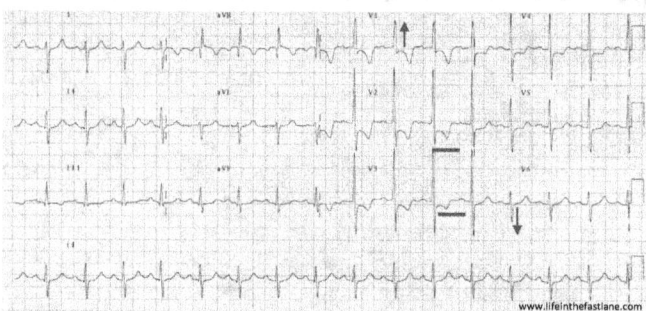

Right ventricular hypertrophy (R.V.H.)..

Ischemic heart disease:

Angina pectoris:

Only 50% of cases get ECG changes..

The ECG abnormality is **ST depression** except in *prinzmetal angina* (*ST elevation*).

Myocardial Infarction:

It is either *ST elevation myocardial infarction* (**STEMI**) or *non-ST elevation myocardial infarction* (**non-STEMI** ' the ST segment is isoelectrical with T wave inversion ')..

Timing:

Acute M.I →ST elevation, hyper-acute T wave..

Recent M.I →ST elevation, T wave inversion..

Old M.I →only Q wave..

Localization: Please, see page 39... & **NEVER** forget it...

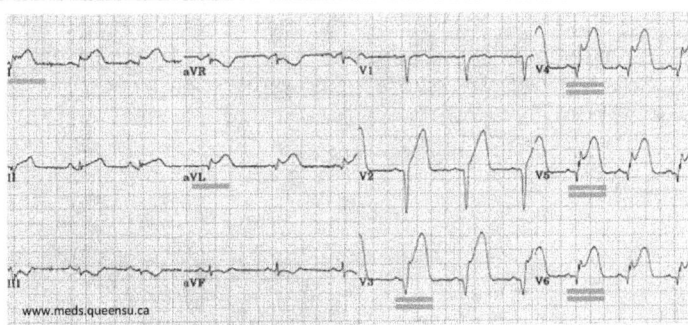

Acute Antero-lateral M.I.

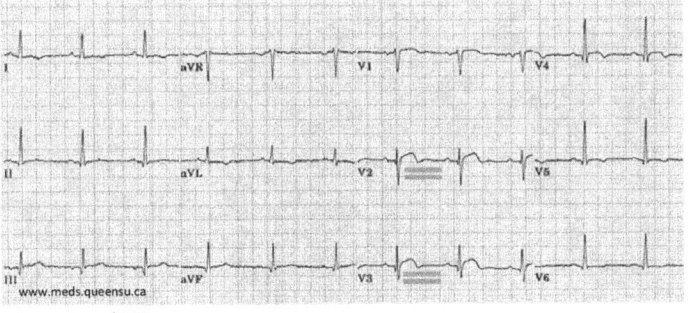

Acute Septal M.I.

2- ECG by M.O.M — ISCHEMIC HEART DISEASE..

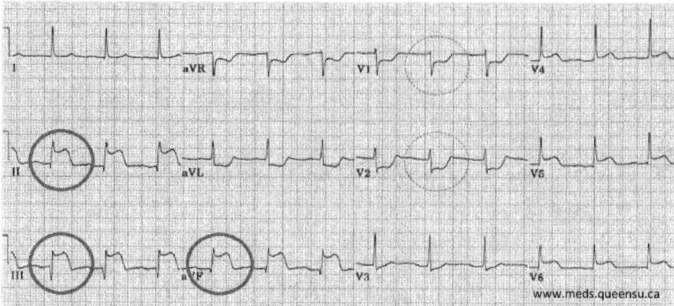

Acute Inferior M.I. associated with ' posterior infarction.. ST segments in leads overlying the posterior region of the heart (V1 and V2) are initially horizontally depressed. As the infarction evolves, lead V1 demonstrates an R wave (which in fact represents a Q wave in reverse).. '

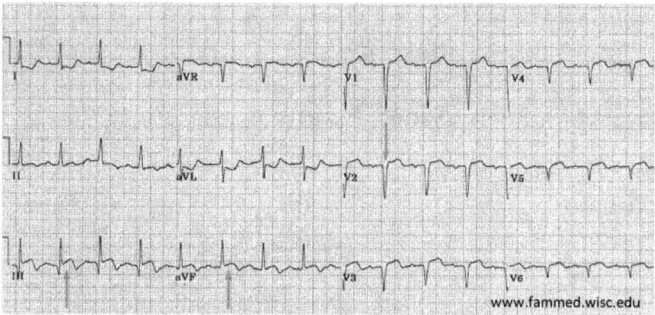

The pathological Q waves seen in V1 - V6 indicate that this patient has had an anterior MI in the past. This patient also has evidence of an acute inferior MI as shown by the ST segment elevation in leads III and aVF.

Heart block:

Atrioventricular block.

1st degree:

P wave & QRS complex →normal

PR interval → prolonged (> 5 □) (> 0.2 sec.)

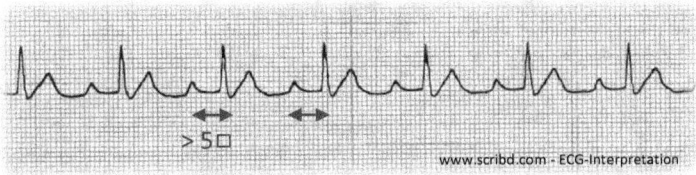

2nd degree:

1- Morbitz type 1: *'Wenckeback phenomena'*

   Progressive PR prolongation then dropped QRS..

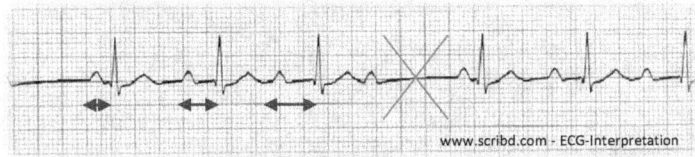

2- Morbitz type 2:

   Sudden drop of QRS, **without prior PR changes..**

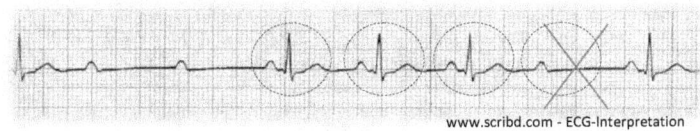

3rd degree:

P is not related to QRS.. *PP rate is regular, BUT is differ from the RR rate (which is also regular)..*

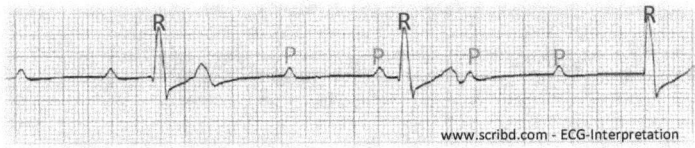

2- ECG by M.O.M — HEART BLOCK..

Note:

The QRS complex in the chest leads shows a *progression* from lead V_1, where it is predominantly **downward**, to lead V_6, where it is predominantly **upward**. The ' transition point ', where the R & S waves are equal, indicates the position of the interventricular septum. So, if the right ventricle is enlarged, and occupies more of the precordium than is normal, the transition point will move from its normal position of leads V_3/V_4 to leads V_4/V_5 or sometimes leads V_5/V_6.

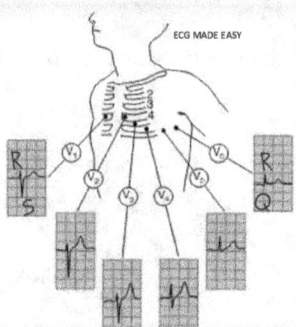

Trick:

You have to know, there is R & S waves in the lead V_1, BUT Q & S waves in V_6 (which is normal septal Q wave) → So, any change in this figure, think about any abnormality like Bundle branch block..

Right bundle branch block (RBBB):

QRS > 0.12 (> 3 □)

In the.. lead V_1 → RSR' wave *(M shape)*.. leads *I* & V_6 → slurred ' broad ' S wave
leads V_{1-3} → T wave inversion

causes : *Idiopathic*, 2° to COPD or 2° to right ventricular pressure overload.

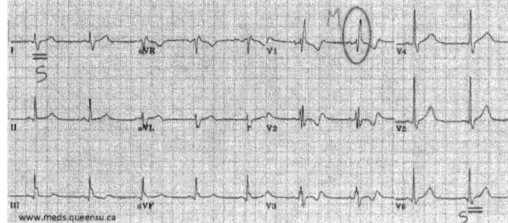

Left bundle branch block (RBBB):

QRS > 0.11 (> 3 □)

In the.. lead I, aVL & V_{5-6} → RSR' wave *(M shape)* and ST depression & T inversion
causes : acute M.I, sever L.V.H., sever aortic stenosis, cardiomyopathy & rarely *Idiopathic*.

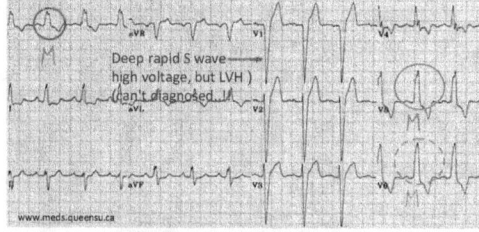

2- ECG by M.O.M — DYSARRHYTHMIA..

Dysarrhythmia:

We depend on the *lead II* strip.. & you have to observe the following:
the rate is *regular, regular irregular, irregular irregular..?*
the P wave & its relation to QRS..
P wave & QRS complex configuration..

Sinus rhythm:
There is P wave for each QRS complex..

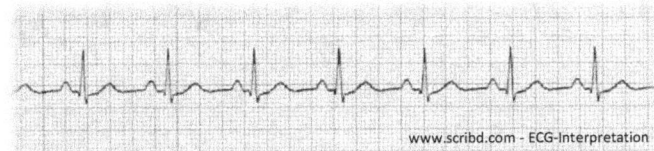

Sinus bradycardia:
P wave for each QRS
PP rate & RR rate < 60 beats/minute
Causes : athletes, hypothyroidism, hypothermia, increase intracranial pressure & inferior M.I.

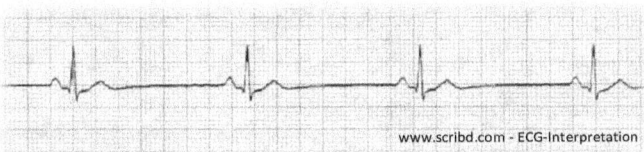

Sinus tachycardia:
P wave for each QRS
PP rate & RR rate >100 beats/minute
Causes : fever, anxiety, exercise, anemia, hyperthyroidism..

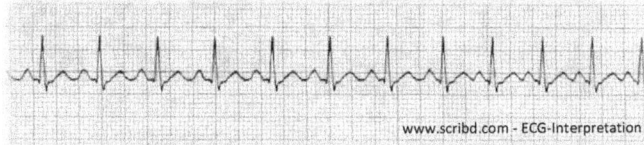

Sinus arrhythmia:
P wave for each QRS
when *longest RR > shortest RR* by *0.16 sec.* (4 □) then sinus arrhythmia is diagnosed..
Causes : normal in infant & young children.. pathological in elderly..

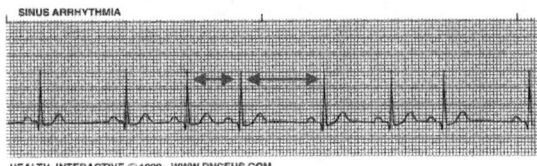

2- ECG by M.O.M — DYSARRHYTHMIA..

Atrial premature contraction (A.P.C.):
Normal ECG → P wave for each QRS
BUT, one P wave is different from previous one &
   the PR interval in this beat is changeable..

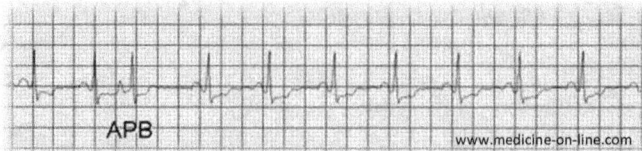

Ventricular premature beat (V.P.B.):
rate → regular
No P wave, wide QRS, T wave is opposite to QRS..
usually followed by compensatory pause..
could be single or multiple.

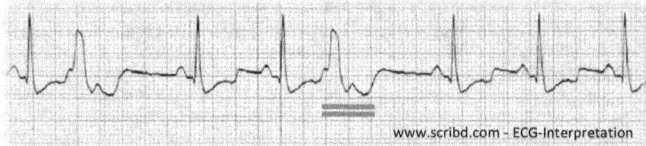

Multifocal atrial tachycardia:
Different *p wave, PR interval, PP & RR rate..*
multiple area of P wave origin.. & usually seen in advance pulmonary disease..

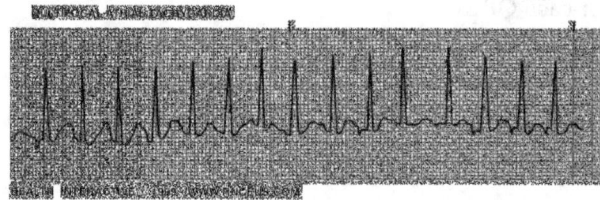

Supra-ventricular tachycardia (S.V.T.):
Heart rate = *160 – 220* b./min.
 regular rhythm..

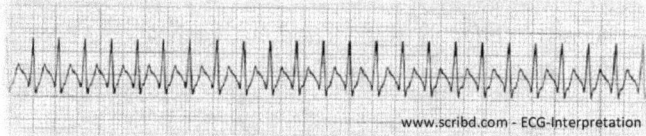

Atrial flutter:
Atrial rate = *250-350* b./min. regular..
PP rate faster than RR rate..
AV block: 2:1, 3:1, 4:1 ... etc
ventricular rate is regular or irregular (depending on the degree of the block)..

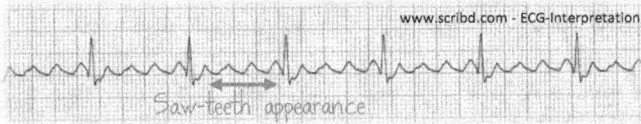

Atrial fibrillation:
rate → completely irregular *' irregular irregular '*..
No P wave, but there is *F wave ' fibrillatory wave '*
Atrial rate = 350-450, ventricular rate is completely irregular..
there is two type of fibrillation: fine and coarse atrial fibrillation..

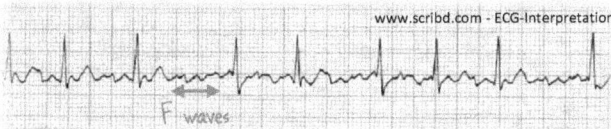

Ventricular tachycardia (V.T.):
No P wave, wide QRS complex, **fast tachycardia**..
usually serious dysarrhythmia → may progress to serious ventricular tachycardia..

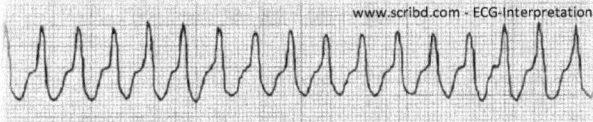

Trick:
Whenever you say *ventricular beat*, this is mean no P wave, wide QRS complex..

Ventricular fibrillation: ' FATAL DYSARRHYTHMIA '
No actual QRS.. rather *bizarre & chaotic undulation* of the base..
there is two type of ventricular fibrillation: fine and coarse fibrillation..

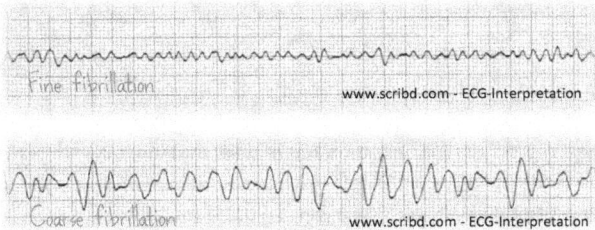

Hyperkalemia & hypokalemia:

Hyperkalemia:

There are *tall, tented, symmetrical T waves* with a narrow base..

The P wave remains normal, as does the QRS complex. the QRS complex broadens and the S wave is widened in leads V3 - V6. This S wave become continuous with the tented T waves and eventually the ST segment disappears.

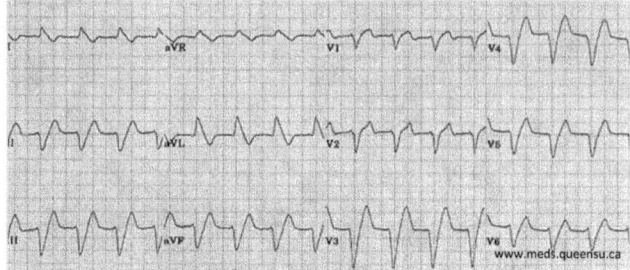

Hypokalemia:

There are *flattening of the T waves*, *U waves* may develop..

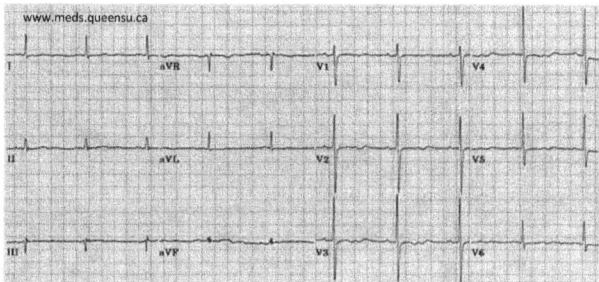

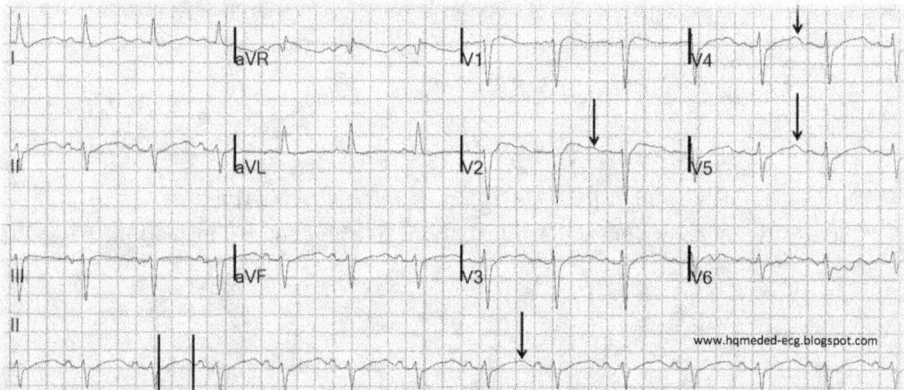

Notice large U-waves (arrows). One is tempted to think that the long hump after the QRS (between the two vertical lines) is the T-wave. Whenever you see this, you should think about both long QT and U-wave. But if you look closely, you see there are 2 bumps, so the second one must be a U-wave.

2- ECG by M.O.M — PERICARDITIS vs. INFARCTION..

Pericarditis vs. Infarction:

Acute pericarditis:

ST segment *elevation, concave* upward....
Usually *diffused*
Start as ST segment elevation → back normal → T wave inversion
No reciprocal changes.. No pathological Q wave
May be PR segment depression ' *very sensitive indicator of acute pericarditis* '..

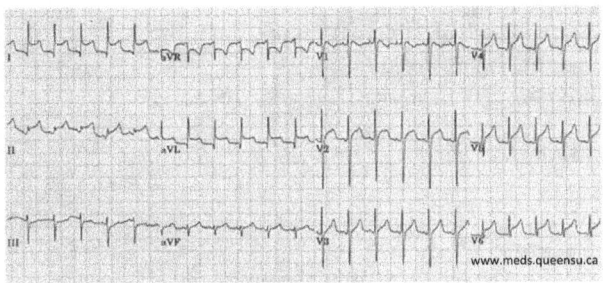

Myocardial infarction:

ST segment *elevation, convex* upward....
Usually *localized*
ST segment elevation, Q wave, T wave inversion may be together..
May be there is reciprocal changes..

Trick:
You can draw an imaginary line between the J point and the apex of the T wave. If the ST segment is below that line, then it's upwardly concave. If it's even with or above that line, then it's upwardly convex, which is suspicious for acute myocardial infarction.

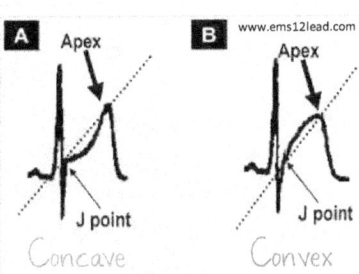

If it helps you to remember, an upwardly concave ST segment makes a "smiley face" (good) and an upwardly convex ST segment makes a "frowny face" (bad).

So, take it easy..
Dr. M.O.M

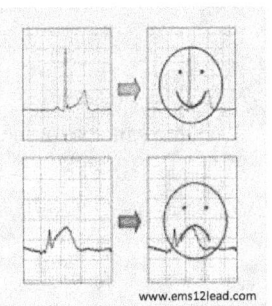

2- ECG by M.O.M — HOW TO READ & REPORT THE ECG??..

How to *read* & *report* the ECG ??

Answer:

It is a **matter of training..**

so, whenever you see an ECG.. read it *systematically* and don't put the diagnosis as an aim.. with time and when you become able to catch a lot of abnormalities then you can easily reach a possible diagnosis..

How to read the ECG ?

1- Start from the labeling.. (NAME, AGE, SEX, EXACT TIME)
2- See the calibration & speed..
3- Make sure normal connection & no dextrocardia

4- Rate & rhythm
5- Axis

6- P wave ' in leads I, II, V_1 '
7- PR interval ' in the lead II strip is the best '

8- QRS complexes & Q wave ' also look for ventricular hypertrophy & bundle branch block '
9- ST segment & T wave

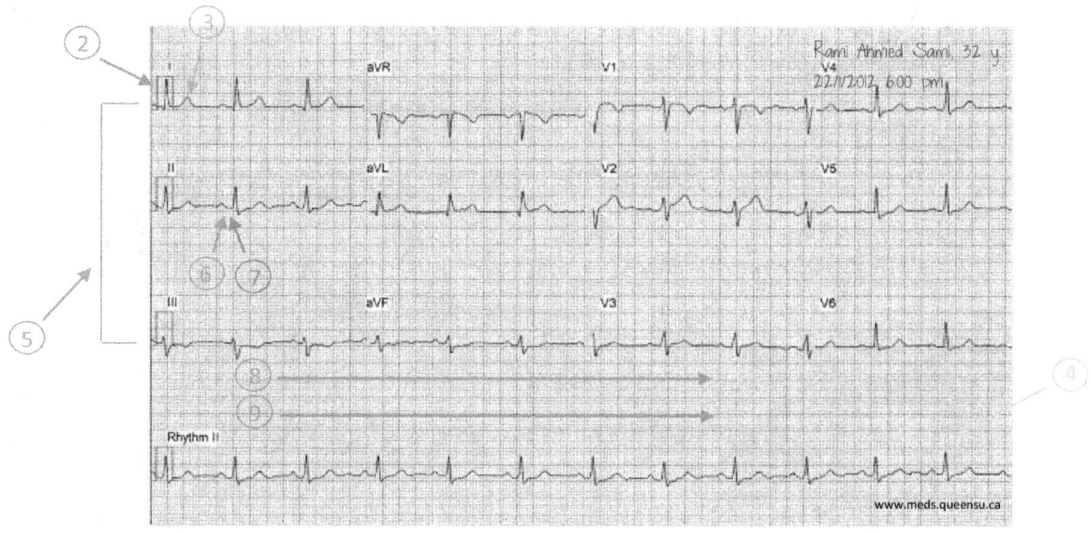

How to report the ECG ?

In the same sequence as for reading the ECG.. but, please don't mention the headlines.. So, *FORGET:*

~~the NAME, AGE, SEX, EXACT TIME, … RATE, RHYTHM….~~ etc.

just like in the reporting of the history..

Inverted P wave in lead I:

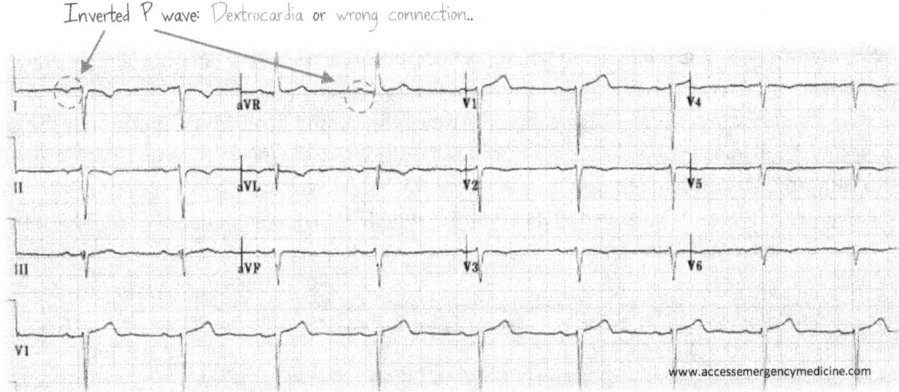

Inverted P wave: Dextrocardia or wrong connection..

Digoxin toxicity:

Digoxin effect refers to the presence on the ECG of:
Down-sloping ST depression with a characteristic *"sagging"* appearance
Flattened, inverted, or biphasic T waves.
Shortened QT interval

The morphology of the QRS complex / ST segment is variously described as either slurred, sagging or scooped and resembling either a reverse tick, hockey stick or (my personal favorite) *'Salvador Dali's moustache'* !

The most common T-wave abnormality is a **biphasic T wave** with an initial negative deflection and terminal positive deflection. This is usually seen in leads with a dominant R wave (e.g. V4-6). The first part of the T wave is typically continuous with the depressed ST segment. The terminal positive deflection may be peaked, or have a prominent U wave superimposed upon it.

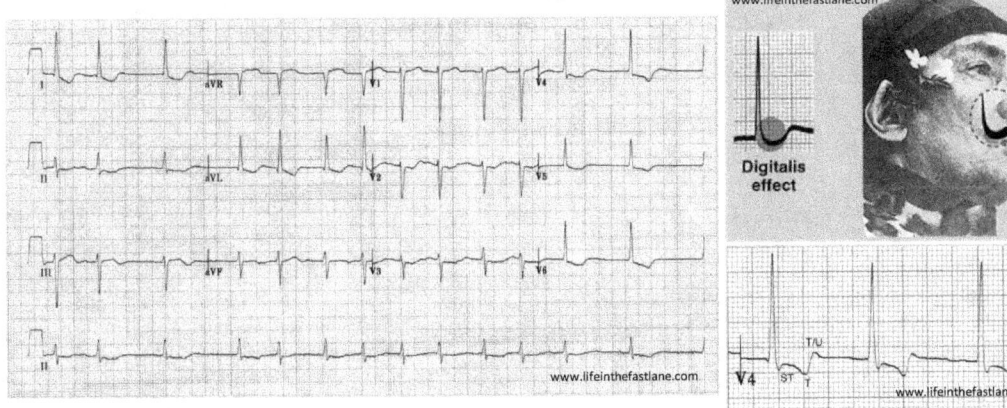

Wolff-Parkinson-White syndrome:

Diagnosis of W.P.W. is based on the ECG interpretation..

PR interval <0.12 seconds, P waves of normal appearance

QRS complex is wide, with a longer duration than 0.12 seconds

The presence of delta waves ' Slow enrollment or thickening of the initial portion of the QRS complex (delta wave) is the most important criterion for diagnosis of Wolff-Parkinson-White syndrome, Delta wave length range between 0.02-0.07 seconds '

Secondary changes of ST segment and T wave, which are showing a opposite direction from the QRS complex and delta wave.

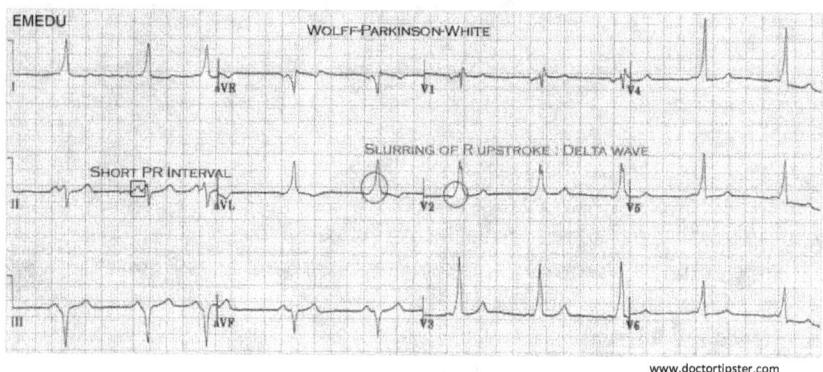

Ventricular asystole:

Simply, there is *NOTHING*..

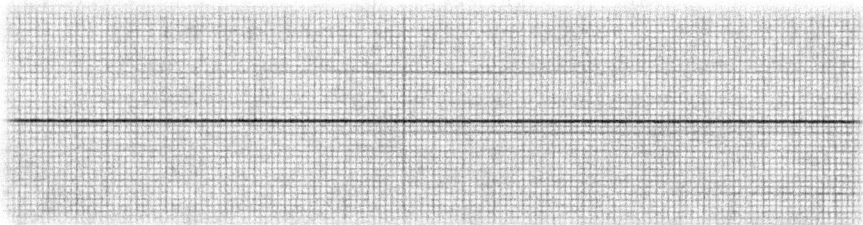

CHAPTER 3

SURGERY

Contents:

HISTORY TAKING
- Pain H_x — 62
- Yellowish discoloration of sclera & skin H_x — 63
- Bleeding per rectum H_x — 64
- Lump or Ulcer H_x — 65
- Goiter H_x — 66
- Breast lump H_x — 67
- Peptic ulcer H_x — 68
- Upper gastrointestinal bleeding H_x — 69
- Gallstone pain H_x — 70
- Gastric outlet obstruction H_x — 70

EXAMINATION
- Ulcer E_x. — 71
- Lump E_x. — 72
- Thyroid status E_x — 73
- Thyroid E_x. — 74
- Hernia E_x. — 75
- Breast E_x. — 77
- Abdominal E_x. — 78
- Post-operative E_x. — 79
- Wound E_x. — 80
- Chest tube E_x. — 81
- Drains E_x. — 82
- Stoma E_x. — 83

PERIPHERAL VASCULAR EXAMINATION
- Lower limb — 84
- Varicose veins — 86
- Upper limb — 87

MEDICAL SKILL LAB
- Per rectum examination — 89
- Nasogastric tube placement — 90
- Foley's catheter insertion — 91
- Cannula insertion — 92
- Chest tube placement — 93
- I.M. injection — 94
- Indications, complications, C.I. & removal ' in brief ' — 95

RADIOLOGY
- How to report ' The chest X-ray ' — 97
- How to report ' The abdominal X-ray ' — 98
- Some of important X-rays & other radiological studies — 99

UROSURGERY
- Genitourinary problems ' H_x taking ' — 101
- Hematuria H_x, pain H_x — 102
- Abdominal E_x — 103
- General E_x related to urosurgery — 103
- Genital E_x — 105
- How to report ' urosurgery radiological studies ' — 106
- Urosurgery - Instruments — 108

3- SURGERY — GENERAL SURGERY ' focus HISTORY TAKING '..

Pain ' history taking ':

Site:

Duration:
Onset: sudden or gradual..

Character/Nature: stabbing, burning, colicky ...etc

Severity: can't walk or do the daily performance..

Radiation/Referral:

Progression: any change in the pain.. ↑↑ or ↓↓ at specific time.. continuous or intermittent..

Aggravating & relieving factors:

Associated symptoms: fever, rigor or if abdominal pain also ask about nausea & vomiting, yellowish discoloration of the skin & sclera, blood in stool....etc

Any previous attack: *very important..*
Urogenital Hx: *very important..*
Menstrual Hx: *very important..*

Drug Hx: alcohol included..

Trick:

First, You have to great the patient, introduce yourself, take permission from the patient.. then start to ask about the demography of the patient (NAME, AGE, SEX..etc.) then the chief complaint & duration, Hx of present illness, review of systems......, past medical past surgical, drug Hx, Family Hx ....etc

So, Focus Hx means you have to concentrate on the chief complaint & related system and mention the other symptoms in brief ' *not in details* '... BUT, you have to mention all the divisions of the Hx which is described in page 2 ..

3- SURGERY — GENERAL SURGERY 'focus HISTORY TAKING'..

Yellowish discoloration of sclera & skin ' history taking ':

Duration:
Onset:

Pallor: ?

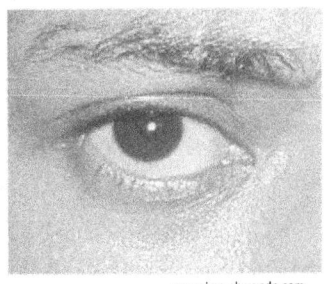

Urine & stool color: dark urine & pale ' clay ' stool..
Color of sclera & skin: lemonade greenish..?

Itching: ?
Pain: *painless jaundice suggest malignancy..*
Associated symptoms: fever & rigor (cholangitis), weight loss

Family Hx:

Past medical Hx: any hemolytic disease, bleeding tendency,

Past surgical Hx: H_x of blood transfusion..

Drug Hx: alcohol, I.V. drug injections.. &
ASNANK (aspirin, sulfa drugs, nitrofurantoin, anti-malarial, nalidixic acid, Vit. K)..

Other: sexual H_x, travel H_x, H_x of shellfish ingestion (Hepatitis A. Virus)..

Trick:
First, You have to great the patient, introduce yourself, take permission from the patient.. then start to ask about the demography of the patient (NAME, AGE, SEX..etc.) then the chief complaint & duration, H_x of present illness, review of systems……. ,past medical past surgical, drug H_x, Family H_x …..etc

So, Focus H_x means you have to concentrate on the chief complaint & related system and mention the other symptoms in brief ' *not in details* '... BUT, you have to mention all the divisions of the Hx which is described in page 2 ..

3- SURGERY — GENERAL SURGERY ' focus HISTORY TAKING '..

Bleeding per rectum ' history taking ':

Duration:
Onset:

Severity: **continuous ?**

During, before or after defecation:

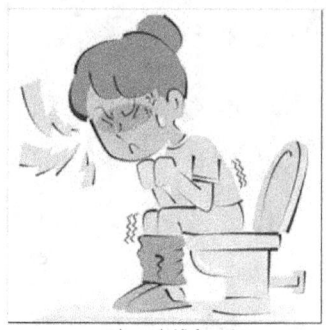
www.hemorrhoidinformationcenter.com

Amount & color of the blood:
Color of the stool:

Alteration in bowel habit:
Tenesmus: *' painful straining without resultant evacuation '*

Pain:
Discharge & itching: **any hemolytic disease, bleeding tendency,**

Weight loss, ↓↓ appetite, pallor:

Family Hx:
Past medical Hx: **previous attack, bleeding disease, another site of bleeding..**

Drug Hx:

Trick:
   First, You have to greet the patient, introduce yourself, take permission from the patient.. then start to ask about the demography of the patient (NAME, AGE, SEX..etc.) then the chief complaint & duration, Hx of present illness, review of systems........ ,past medical past surgical, drug Hx, Family Hx ....etc

   So, Focus Hx means you have to concentrate on the chief complaint & related system and mention the other symptoms in brief *' not in details '*... BUT, you have to mention all the divisions of the Hx which is described in page 2 ..

3- SURGERY — GENERAL SURGERY ' focus HISTORY TAKING '..

Lump or Ulcer ' history taking ':

Site & Duration:

1st symptom ' brought it to the patient notice ':
like pain, bleeding, purulent discharge, foul smell,
notice by other person or at bathroom.. etc

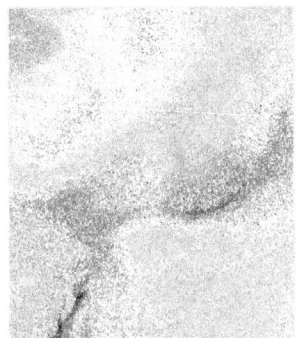
www.greensboroearnosethroat.com

Other symptoms:
interfere with walking, eating or daily activity
(in Lump: interfere with movement, respiration
or swelling & any redness or hotness)

Progression: size, shape & discharge..

Persistent: healed or disappeared ??

Other or previous lump or ulcer:

Cause: any injury or systemic disease..etc

Trick:

First, You have to great the patient, introduce yourself, take permission from the patient.. then start to ask about the demography of the patient (NAME, AGE, SEX..etc.) then the chief complaint & duration, H_x of present illness, review of systems....... ,past medical past surgical, drug H_x, Family H_x ....etc

So, Focus H_x means you have to concentrate on the chief complaint & related system and mention the other symptoms in brief ' not in details '.. BUT, you have to mention all the divisions of the Hx which is described in page 2 ..

3- SURGERY — GENERAL SURGERY 'focus HISTORY TAKING'..

Goiter ' history taking ':

H$_x$ OF LUMP: *as mention in previous page..*

Pain, discomfort on swallowing, shortness of breath, stridor, Horsiness, or cosmoses:

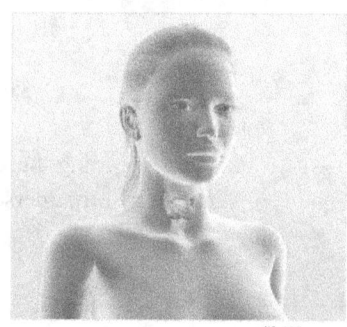

Eye: protruding, difficulty in closure, pain, double vision or swelling of conjunctiva..

Nervous: nervousness, insomnia or irritability

Cardiovascular: palpitation & shortness of breath on exertion

G.I.T.: ↑↑ appetite + ↓↓ weight *(or the reverse)*.. early morning diarrhea or constipation..

Preference: hot (or cold) weather intolerance..

Amenorrhea & menorrhagia in ♀, libido & impotence in ♂:

Change in face appearance, skin or hair:

Drug H$_x$: radioiodine R$_x$ included..

Past surgical H$_x$: any previous thyroid surgery

Trick:

First, You have to great the patient, introduce yourself, take permission from the patient.. then start to ask about the demography of the patient (NAME, AGE, SEX..etc.) then the chief complaint & duration, H$_x$ of present illness, review of systems....... ,past medical past surgical, drug H$_x$, Family H$_x$ ....etc

So, Focus H$_x$ means you have to concentrate on the chief complaint & related system and mention the other symptoms in brief ' not in details '.. BUT, you have to mention all the divisions of the Hx which is described in page 2 ..

3- SURGERY — GENERAL SURGERY ' focus HISTORY TAKING '..

Breast lump ' history taking ':

Hx OF LUMP: *as mention in previous page..*

Pain, size (change with menstrual cycle):

Breast size & shape changes:
Skin & nipple changes:

Fever, weight loss, bone or abdominal pain:
Arm swelling, axillary lump, breathlessness, yellowish discoloration of sclera & headache:

Previous radiation or surgery:

Menstrual Hx: menarche, menopause, contraceptive pills, hormone replacement ..etc
Obstetric Hx: parity

Breast feeding & if there are any complications, previous mammography or screening:

Family Hx: breast, bowel & ovarian CA..

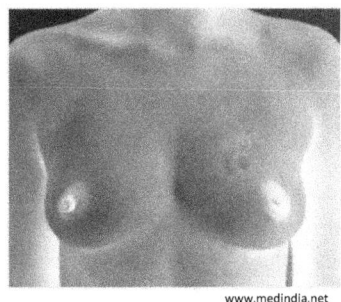

Trick:

    First, You have to great the patient, introduce yourself, take permission from the patient.. then start to ask about the demography of the patient (NAME, AGE, SEX..etc.) then the chief complaint & duration, Hx of present illness, review of systems......., past medical past surgical, drug Hx, Family Hx ....etc

    So, Focus Hx means you have to concentrate on the chief complaint & related system and mention the other symptoms in brief *' not in details '*... BUT, you have to mention all the divisions of the Hx which is described in page 2 ..

3- SURGERY — GENERAL SURGERY ' focus HISTORY TAKING '..

Peptic ulcer ' history taking ':

Onset & duration:

Pain Hx:

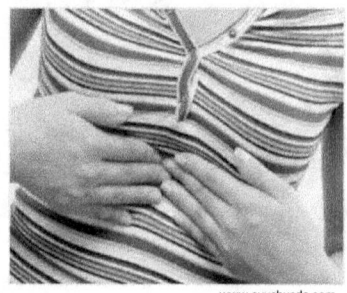
www.ayushveda.com

    Some of the expected answer:
- epigastric pain.. radiated to the back..
- intermitted, last from weeks to months with pain free interval
- may eat or (avoid eating) to relieve pain
- more in spring & autumn seasons

Vomiting: **absent unless pyloric stenosis**

Alteration in weight:

Bleeding: **upper GIT bleeding or lower GIT bleeding** (malaena)

Pallor:

Complication: bleeding, perforation & pyloric stenosis symptoms

Drug Hx: **aspirin, NSAID, steroid, food poisoning, burn or major surgery..**

Trick:

    First, You have to greet the patient, introduce yourself, take permission from the patient.. then start to ask about the demography of the patient (NAME, AGE, SEX..etc.) then the chief complaint & duration, Hx of present illness, review of systems......., past medical past surgical, drug Hx, Family Hx .....etc

    So, Focus Hx means you have to concentrate on the chief complaint & related system and mention the other symptoms in brief ' not in details '... BUT, you have to mention all the divisions of the Hx which is described in page 2 ..

3- SURGERY — GENERAL SURGERY ' focus HISTORY TAKING '..

Upper Gastrointestinal bleeding ' history taking ':

Onset & duration:

Severity: continuous ?

Color of blood: fresh, bright red or coffee ground
Color of stool: black, terry stool (malaena)

Amount:

Preceding by intense retching:

Weight loss, pallor & pain:

Past medical Hx: previous attack, any liver disease (varices) or bleeding tendency

Drug Hx: aspirin, warfarin..

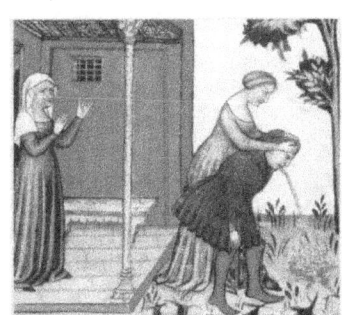

www.stemlyns.files.wordpress.com

Trick:
   First, You have to great the patient, introduce yourself, take permission from the patient.. then start to ask about the demography of the patient (NAME, AGE, SEX..etc.) then the chief complaint & duration, Hx of present illness, review of systems......., past medical past surgical, drug Hx, Family Hx ....etc

   So, Focus Hx means you have to concentrate on the chief complaint & related system and mention the other symptoms in brief ' not in details '.. BUT, you have to mention all the divisions of the Hx which is described in page 2 ..

3- SURGERY — GENERAL SURGERY ' focus HISTORY TAKING '..

Gallstone pain ' history taking ':

Some of the expected answer:
- right upper quadrant pain
- sever, last from minutes to hours
- colicky or dull & constant
- radiated to the back or chest, referred to right shoulder tip
- dyspepsia, hurt-burn & flatulence
- food intolerance esp. fatty food..
- does it started during night or awaken the patient..?
- alteration in bowel habit..

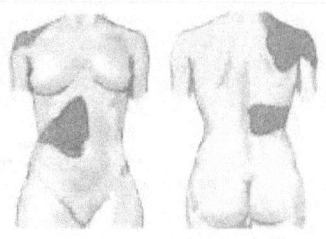
www.curezone.com

Gastric outlet obstruction ' history taking ':

Some of the expected answer:
- H_x of longstanding peptic ulcer
- Unremitting pain
- Unpleasant vomiting, without bile
- *Projectile* vomiting
- Weight loss, unwell, dehydrated ..etc

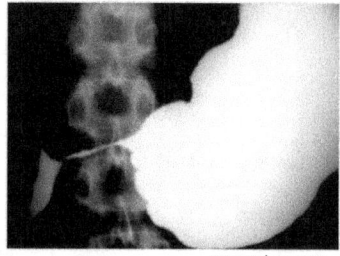
www.medscape.com

Trick:

First, You have to great the patient, introduce yourself, take permission from the patient.. then start to ask about the demography of the patient (NAME, AGE, SEX..etc.) then the chief complaint & duration, H_x of present illness, review of systems....... ,past medical past surgical, drug H_x, Family H_x .....etc

So, Focus H_x means you have to concentrate on the chief complaint & related system and mention the other symptoms in brief ' not in details '... BUT, you have to mention all the divisions of the Hx which is described in page 2 ..

3- SURGERY — ULCER examination..

Ulcer examination:

First: greet the patient,

introduce yourself,

take permission for examination,

hand washing,

make sure patient privacy,

good exposure

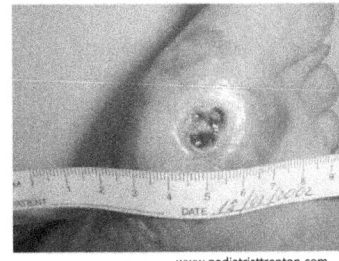

www.podiatristtrenton.com

Trick: If there is dressing, you have to remove & describe it (clean, soiled with blood..etc)..

LOCAL: ' the ulcer '

Inspection: site, size, shape, color, discharge *(wound & dressing)* , *floor, depth, edge..*
(3S + CD + *the dimensions..*)

what you see

Palpation: *ask if he has any pain*, temperature, tenderness, base *(wear gloves , soft or indurated ?)..*

what you feel

Surrounding & local tissue:

Trick: You have to see between the fingers & elevate the leg to see the pressure areas.. looking for ischmec changes..

REGIONAL: ' the lower limb ' for example..

hair loss, swelling, skin lesions, amputation, dilated veins,

temperature, capillary refilling, pulses(dorsalis pedis, ant. tibial, post. tibial, popliteal, femoral)

lymph nodes,

sensation, movement of the joint (motor)..

GENERAL: in diabetic foot for example..

weight loss, vital signs (postural hypotension),

eye examination, boil in the neck..

At the end: you can suggest to take a bacteriological swab
cover the patient, thank him..

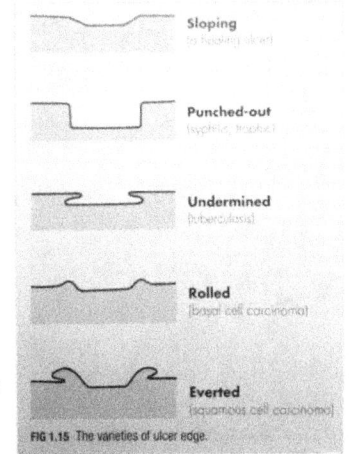

FIG 1.15 The varieties of ulcer edge.

Browse's introduction to the symptoms & signs of surgical diseases..

3- SURGERY — LUMP examination..

Lump examination:

First: greet the patient,

introduce yourself,

take permission for examination,

hand washing & warming,

make sure patient privacy,

good exposure

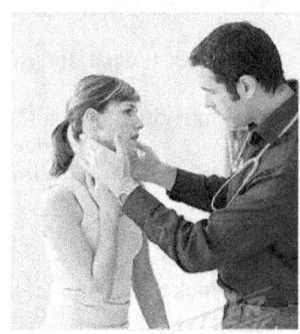

LOCAL: ' the lump'

Inspection: site, size, shape, surface, color, discharge, *edge..*
(4S + CD + *edge..*)

Palpation: *ask if he has any pain*, temperature, tenderness,

content *(consistency)*, mobility, edge,

fixation *(may need technique to contract the muscle)* & tethering (to skin),

compressibility & reducibility,

pulsation, thrill, fluctuation,

trans- illumination

Trick: If the lump is suspected hernia then you have to ask the patient to cough in inspection & palpation..

Percussion:

Auscultation:

Surrounding & local tissue:

REGIONAL: vascular, nervous, lymph nodes examination..

GENERAL:

At the end: cover the patient, thank him..

3- SURGERY — THYROID examination..

Thyroid status examination:

General look: agitation, nervousness, lethargy

Hand: sweating, redness & temperature,

clubbing *(thyroid achropathy)*, onycholysis,

palmer erythema, *tremor (fine fast)*,

radial pulse *(sleeping pulse is the best..!!)*

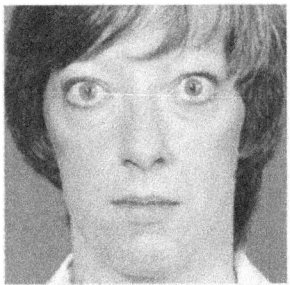
www.the-hospitalist.org

Head: *' apart from the eye.. '*

hair, malar flush, speech, Horner's syndrome &

ask him to open his mouth to see the tonsils and lingual glands..

Eyes: lid retraction, lid lag, forehead wrinkling, *exophthalmus (by Naffziger's method)*,

ophthalmoplagia & convergence, chemosis..

Then do complete thyroid examination..

Leg: ankle reflex (delayed relaxation), myxoedema, proximal myopathy..

3- SURGERY   THYROID examination..

Thyroid examination:

Trick: the examination with the patient sitting on a chair..

First: greet the patient,

introduce yourself,

take permission for examination,

hand washing & warming,

make sure patient privacy,

good exposure

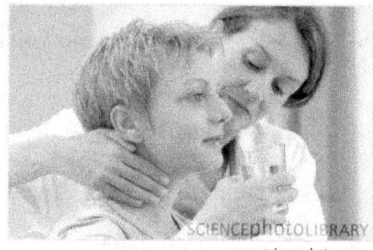

Trick: Pemberto's test.. ask the patient to elevate her hands & flex her neck for 1 min. (if there is cyanosis, stridor or congestion → means retrosternal goiter)..

LOCAL: ' the Goiter '

Inspection: ask the patient to **swallow sip of water, put the tongue outside..**

  describe it as a LUMP *(mention in previous page)*,
  (4S + CD + *edge*..)

don't forget to look for dilated veins, scar or visible pulsation..

Palpation: from **front** as any LUMP (temperature & tenderness), trachea, thyroid cartilage..

from **the back..** ' *the technique is very important.. '*

- put your two thumbs on the ligamintum nuchae & your 2 index fingers below the mandible & feel the gland by the other fingers..

- try to relax the neck muscles and press one lobe while palpating the other..

now again, ask the patient to **swallow sip of water, put the tongue outside..**

then describe it as any LUMP..

  don't forget the carotid pulse for (Berry's sign) & L.N.

Percussion: on the lower part of the gland, clavicles, sternum & upper chest wall.. ' *to exclude retrosternal goiter.. '*

Auscultation: for bruit & machinery murmur..

REGIONAL: shoulders, axilla (ask her to elevate her arms), upper arm, head & mouth..

GENERAL: *thyroid status ' mentioned in previous page '..*

At the end: cover the patient, thank him..

3- SURGERY — HERNIA examination..

Hernia examination:

The order is either:
- examine the hernia,
- abdominal examination or
- examine the scar..

Inguinal hernia examination must be in 2 postion:
- supine &
- standing ' *the best* '..

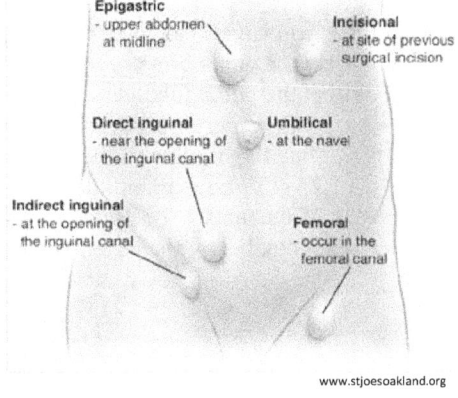

First: greet the patient,

introduce yourself,

take permission for examination,

hand washing & warming,

make sure patient privacy,

good exposure

Trick: You have to stand beside the patient (at the same side of the examined area & at the same level), examine by one hand and support his buttock by other hand..

LOCAL: ' the Hernia '

Inspection: describe it as a LUMP, but don't forget to ask the patient to COUGH..
(4S + CD + *edge*..)

note: indirect inguinal hernia → pyriform in shape, the direct → globular..
don't forget to look for visible pulsation & penis deviation *(if it is large)*..

Palpation: describe it as a LUMP *(mentioned before)*,
but, don't forget to ask the patient to COUGH..
in large inguinal hernia, make sure whether it *reaches the scrotum or not.. & can get above the testis or not..*

Percussion:

Auscultation:

Special tests: to differentiate between direct, indirect & femoral hernias.. **(see next page)**

REGIONAL: the abdomen, scrotum, P.R.

GENERAL: the chest examination is also important..

At the end: cover the patient, thank him..

3- SURGERY   HERNIA examination..

SPECIAL TESTS:

First, you have to localize the anatomy..
- feel the pubic bone
- feel the pubic tubercle
- feel the anterior superior iliac spine
- define the midline of the inguinal ligament
- 1.25 cm. above pubic tubercle → superficial inguinal ring
  1.25 cm. above the middle of inguinal ligament → deep inguinal ring
  2.5 cm. below the middle of inguinal ligament → femoral ring

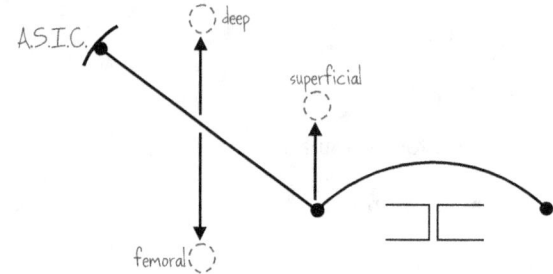

Remember, you have to ask the patient if he can *reduce the hernia..* if he can't → then you have to reduce it by **taxis** technique (first, make sure there are no contraindication for this technique)..

3 fingers test: *thumb* on → **deep** ing. ring → feel *indirect* inguinal hernia

index on → **superficial** ing. ring → feel *direct* inguinal hernia

middle finger on → **femoral** ring → feel *femoral* hernia

Occlusion test: reduce the hernia.. close the deep inguinal ring.. then ask the patient to cough..

if there is *no swelling* in the superficial ring → the hernia is *indirect..*

if there is *swelling* in the superficial ring → the hernia is *direct..*

invagination test: painful (forbidden nowadays..)

3- SURGERY — BREAST examination..

Breast examination:

breast examination must be in 2 positions:
- supine &
- sitting position..

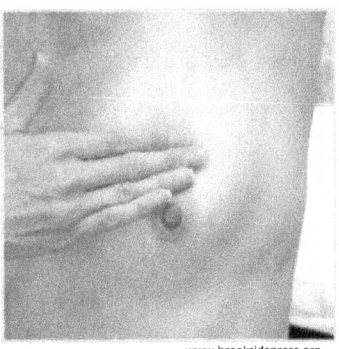
www.brooksidepress.org.

First: greet the patient,

introduce yourself,

take permission for examination,

hand washing & warming,

make sure patient privacy,

good exposure *' above the waist '*

LOCAL: ' the Breast '

Trick: You can use the palm of the hand, palmer surface of the fingers or the thumb & fingers ' more sensitive '. for examination of the breast..

Inspection: size, symmetry, contour..

skin *(color, puckering, ulceration, thickening, nodularity, peau d'orange)*

dilated veins, scar

areola, nipple *' destruction, depression, discoloration, displacement, deviation, discharge, duplication '*

Palpation: ask the patient to localize the lump if present.. examine the normal breast first..

examine all the breast *' 4 quadrants + tail + areola + nipple '*

if there is a LUMP → examine it as mentioned in previous page..

if retracted nipple → try to reverse it.. If there is discharge → take swab

if you want to see the relation to the muscles → ask the patient to put her hands & press on the hips *' if the lump become not mobile → fixed, mobile → tethering '*

REGIONAL: axilla, arm,
supraclavicular fossa *' ask her to raise her hands above the head.. '*

GENERAL: chest, abdomen, P.R., P.V., lumbar spine, nervous system

At the end: cover the patient, thank her..

Trick: Most common involved quadrant by CA.

3- SURGERY — ABDOMINAL examination..

Abdominal examination:

Described previously in details *in chapter ' 1 '..*
See page 23 ..

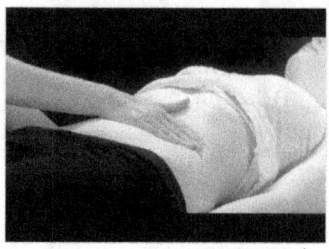

Trick:

If you see a lump in the abdomen (para-umbilical hernia for example) *then examine it in the same sequence with the abdomen..*

In other words, when you do inspection to the abdomen, do complete inspection to the lump (as mentioned before) & so on..

Trick:

You have to ask the patient to COUGH.
Never ever.. forget this point..

Trick:

McBurney's point !.. is the name given to the point over the right side of the abdomen that is one-third of the distance from the anterior superior iliac spine[3] to the umbilicus[2]..

its benefits: *site of auscultation*
site of grid iron incision
site of maximum pain in appendicitis
base of appendix

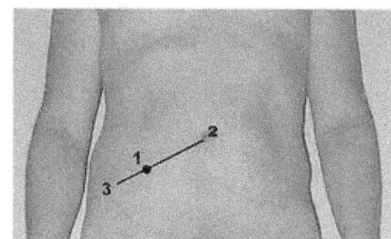

3- SURGERY — POST-OPERATIVE examination..

Post-operative examination:

First: greet the patient,

introduce yourself,

take permission for examination,

hand washing & warming,

make sure patient privacy,

good exposure ' *when needed* '.

ask the patient if he has any *pain*..

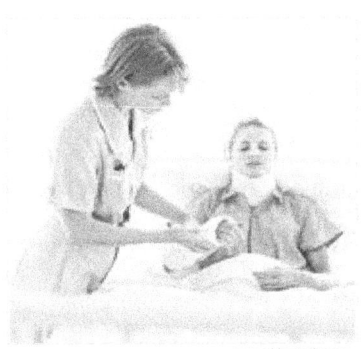

General look: look ill, well, proper sitting of the patient in the bed ..etc

Hand: pallor, cyanosis

Vital signs: *radial pulse*, temperature, blood pressure, respiratory rate

Cannula & I.V. fluid or blood: describe the color of cannula & type of fluid..etc

Head & mouth: pallor, cyanosis, dry or wet tongue *(hydration state)*

Chest: from the anterior & from the back *(do only auscultation if there is no time in exam..)*

Operative site: *dressing, wound*, sutures, *drains* (content, kink or functioning, blockage..etc)

Abdomen: do complete examination to the abdomen *(the inspection & auscultation are the most important)..*

Urine output: see if he has Foley's catheter

Legs: any swelling, *D.V.T. signs*, *edema* & don't forget the pressure areas..

Other less important points:

make sure the histopathology was send to the LAB.. if the patient need blood..
see the operative note of the surgeon, any specific I_x or chart..

ask about.. bowel motion, pass flatus, pass urine, walking after operation, thirst..

give him advices about diet, movement..etc..

At the end: cover the patient, thank him..

3- SURGERY — WOUND examination..

Wound examination:

is just like the *ULCER* examination..

BUT, there are some different point you have to mention. The wound examination is part from post-operative examination ' as you see, was mentioned at the ***operative site*** examination '..

So, *it is very important topic.*

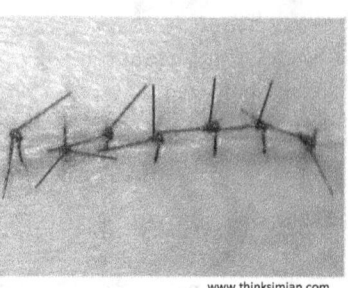

Dressing: describe it (clean, soiled with blood..etc)

Site: anatomical site + name of incision

Size, shape & margin:

Signs of infection: redness, discharge & color of surrounding skin

Color: red (new, <6 mo.), white (healed, > 6mo.)
Hypertrophied or keloid :

Sutures: interrupted, continuous..etc & suture material

Floor, discharge:

Cough: to see if there is any hernia.. *' don't do this step if the wound is open '..*

Surrounding tenderness, temperature & crepitation :

Lymph node:

Mention at the end: *the wound is clean or dirty & infected..etc*

I suggest to take swab from the wound

3- SURGERY — CHEST TUBE examination..

Chest tube examination:

First: greet the patient,

introduce yourself,

take permission for examination,

hand washing & warming,

ask the patient if there is any pain,

make sure patient privacy,

good exposure

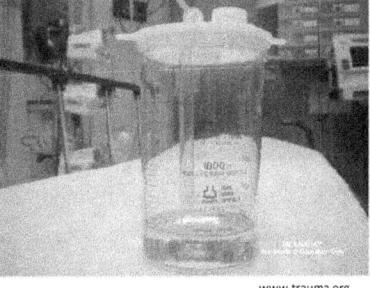
www.trauma.org

Inspection: Name of the drain + name of each part

Site of insertion

Tissue surrounding the insertion site (any infection ?)

Under water seal position to the patient

Amount, color, type of fluid & if there is any clots

Obstruction, kink, displacement

Check the function of the tube
(the fluid in the tube is move with respiration & coughing)

Auscultation: Anterior auscultation

Lateral auscultation

Posterior auscultation

Indication of removal: Medical → the patient is well & normal breathing sounds
Mechanical → drain NOTHING..
By X-ray → full expansion of the lung

At the end: cover the patient, thank him..

3- SURGERY — DRAINS examination..

Drains examination:

The examination of closed *drains, chest tube, NG-tube, Foley's catheter..etc* is the same..

Drains examination is part from post-operative examination ' as you see, was mentioned at the ***operative site*** examination '. So, *it is very important topic.*

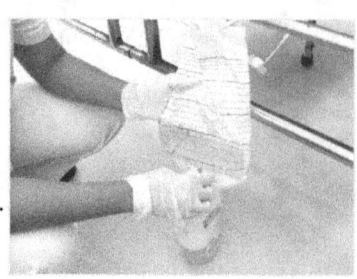

Name: name of the drain + name of each part (collecting bag, tube ..etc)

Site:

Active or passive, Open or closed:

Amount, color, type of fluid & if there is any clots:

Obstruction, kink, displacement:

Functioning or not: *(for example.. ask the patient to cough in chest tube)*

3- SURGERY — STOMA examination..

Stoma examination:

Must be in 3 positions:
- supine,
- sitting &
- standing position..

First: greet the patient,

introduce yourself,

take permission for examination,

hand washing,

make sure patient privacy,

good exposure

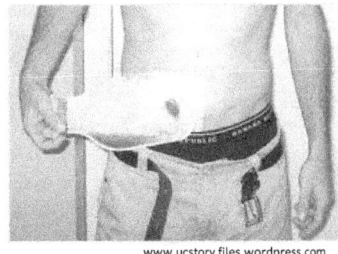

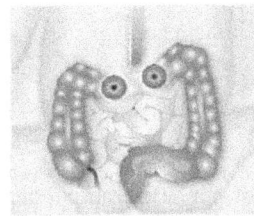

Double barrel stoma   Loop stoma   www.convatec.com.au

LOCAL: ' the Stoma '

Inspection: **site..** any quadrant, well sited (away from bony prominence, scar, skin folds)

scar

content.. liquid, formed feces or urine

morphology.. spouted (ileostomy), flesh (colostomy)..

lumen.. single (end) or double (loop)

identify afferent (stool, flauts, large, cephalic),

efferent (mucus, smaller, caudally)

presence of a bridge → newly formed stoma

ischemia, necrosis, ulceration or stenosis

surrounding skin **excoriation & erythema** (in ileostomy)

prolapsed or **parastomal hernia** (*ask the patient to cough*)

open the bag

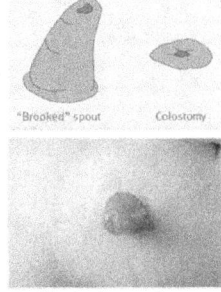

spout (ileostomy) – www. dansac.com

Palpation: temperature & tenderness

digital examination (*wear a glove*.. insert your finger →for patency, stenosis & no. of lumens)

Illumination: to see the mucosa

REGIONAL: abdomen, inspect the perineum for (scar & anal opening) & L.N examination..

GENERAL:

At the end: close the bag, cover the patient & thank him..

3- SURGERY — PERIPHERAL VASCULAR examination..

Lower limb - Peripheral vascular examination:

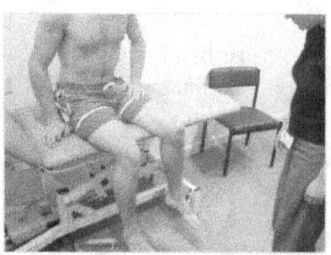

First: greet the patient,

introduce yourself,

take permission for examination,

hand washing,

make sure patient privacy,

ask the patient if there is any pain,

good exposure

Inspection: color of skin, hair distribution, muscle wasting, gangrene *(line of demarcation, wet or dry, any skip area or blebs)*, amputation, scar, swelling, dilated veins & guttering of the vessels

nail changes, if there is an ulcer you have describe it..

don't forget to examine between the fingers, pressure areas *& the groin*

Palpation: *asked him, if he has any pain..* temperature, tenderness & crepitations

edema & signs of D.V.T.,

capillary refill, dorsalis pedis, ant. tibial, post. tibial, popliteal, femoral pulses,

lymph nodes & nervous examination

Auscultation: abdominal aorta bruit, femoral artery bruit, adductor canal bruit

Percussion: sensory *(light touch & pin prick)* , motor

Percussion: over the varicose veins *' tap test '*

Special tests: Burger's test, tourniquet test, Perthe's test, capillary filling time, tap test

*(for more details.. **see next page**)*

At the end: cover the patient & thank him..

3- SURGERY — PERIPHERAL VASCULAR examination..

SPECIAL TESTS – LOWER LIMB:

Burger's test: ask the patient to elevate his leg,
observe at which angle it will become pale,
if the angle < 20° → sever ischemia

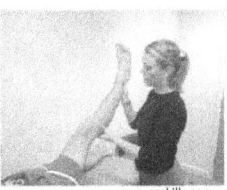

Tourniquet test: elevate the leg 30° & empty the veins..
occlude the saphenous opening by a tourniquet & ask the patient to stand..
then observe the veins…

(if the veins are controlled → the incompetence is above the tourniquet)
(if not… (i.e. rapid refilling) → the incompetence is below the tourniquet)

Perthe's test: empty the veins,
place a tourniquet & ask the patient to stand on their toes..

(if there is pain or dilatation of the veins → D.V.T.)

Capillary filling time: ask the patient to elevate his leg till it become pale,
ask him to hang his legs over the sides of the bed
count the time till it become congested (blue)..

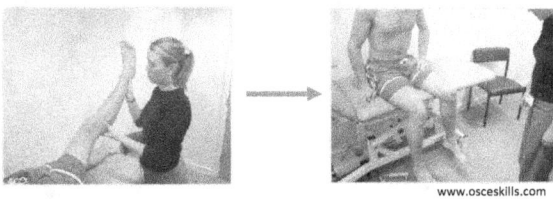

3- SURGERY — PERIPHERAL VASCULAR examination..

Varicose veins:

You have to describe the varicose vein in details whenever you see it during the peripheral vascular examination..

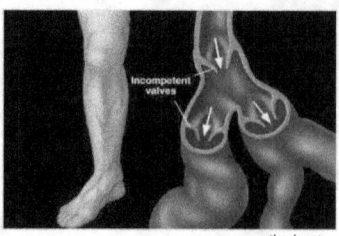

Inspection: it is long or short saphenous vein..?
- long → *from anterio-medial to the malleolus & upward till saphenous opening*
- short → *from the posterior aspect of the calve to the popliteal fossa*
- any blow out (small bulging of veins)
- saphena varix → if present ask the patient to cough to see cough impulse
- elevate the leg → if disappear (incompetence)
  if not (thrombosis)
- Morrissey's test → ask the patient to elevate the leg then ask him to cough look for any bulging & veins impulse

Palpation: temperature & tenderness (thrombophlebitis)
palpate the saphena varix

Percussion: over the various veins ' tap test '

General examination: inguinal L.N., abdomen, scrotum for varicocele & hemorrhoids

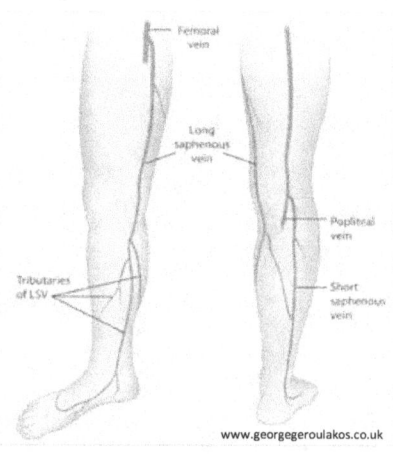

3- SURGERY — PERIPHERAL VASCULAR examination..

Upper limb - Peripheral vascular examination:

First: greet the patient,
introduce yourself,
take permission for examination,
hand washing,
make sure patient privacy,
good exposure

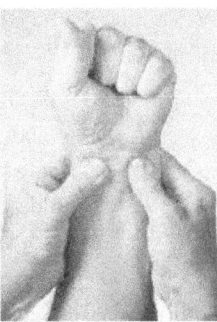
Allen's test — www.kmle.co.kr

Inspection: color of skin, hair distribution, muscle wasting, gangrene *(line of demarcation, wet or dry, any skip area or blebs)*, amputation, scar, swelling, dilated veins, nail changes, pulp atrophy, cyanosis, pallor, if there is an ulcer you have describe it..

Palpation: *asked him, if he has any pain..* temperature, tenderness & crepitations
capillary refill, radial pulse, ulner & brachial pulse, B.P.
axillary artery in axilla, subclavian a., carotid artery & superficial temporal a.,
lymph nodes & nervous examination,
cervical rib..

Auscultation: on supraclavicular, infraclavicular, carotid artery or any abnormal vascular area..

Special tests: Adson's test, elevated arm stress test, Allen's test, Reynaud's phenomenon,
Ankle brachial pressure index..

At the end: cover the patient & thank him..

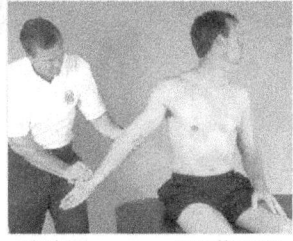
Adson's test — www.mhhe.com11

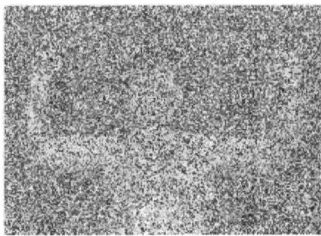
elevated arm stress test — www.cfs9.tistory.com

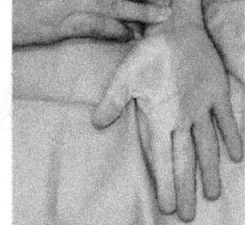
+ve Allen's test — www.2.bp.blogspot.com

3- SURGERY — PERIPHERAL VASCULAR examination..

SPECIAL TESTS -- UPPER LIMB:

Adson's test: The examiner palpates the radial pulse while moving the upper extremity in abduction, extension, and external rotation. The patient then is asked to rotate his head toward the involved side while taking a deep breath and holding it. A positive exam will result in a diminished or absent radial pulse.

Elevated arm stress test: It is performed by having the patient put both arms in the 90° abduction–external rotation position, with the shoulders and elbows in the frontal plane of the chest. The patient is then instructed to open and close the hands slowly over a 3-minute period.

Allen's test:

- The hand is elevated and the patient is asked to make a fist for about 30 seconds.
- Pressure is applied over the ulnar and the radial arteries so as to occlude both of them.
- Still elevated, the hand is then opened. It should appear blanched (pallor can be observed at the finger nails).
- Ulnar pressure is released and the color should return in 7 seconds.
- then do the same step but release the radial pressure.

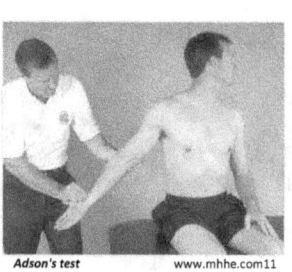

Adson's test   www.mhhe.com11

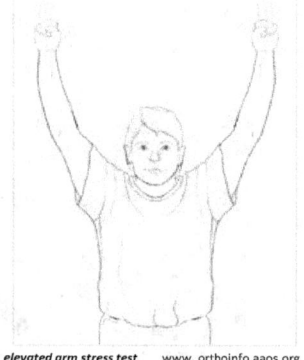

elevated arm stress test   www.orthoinfo.aaos.org

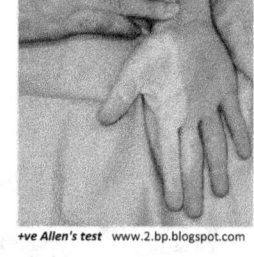

+ve Allen's test   www.2.bp.blogspot.com

3- SURGERY — MEDICAL SKILL LAB..

Per rectal examination:

There are 3 positions for examination:
- left lateral (*Sim's*) position,
- knee-elbow or
- dorsal position..

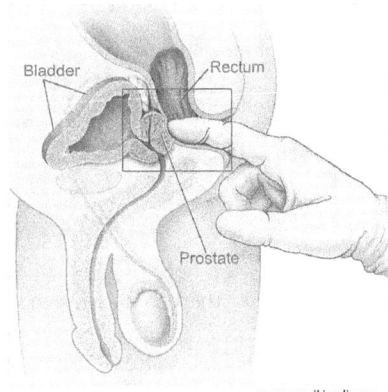
www.en.wikipedia.org

First: greet the patient,

introduce yourself,

take permission for examination,

hand washing,

make sure patient privacy,

good exposure

Inspection: ulcer,

hemorrhoids, fissure, skin tag,

prolapsed, pus, fistula,

bed sore..

Palpation: wear a glove, put lubricant on your index finger, do massage for the external sphincter then introduce your finger..

tenderness, hardness, swelling & tone of the external sphincter,

prostate (size & consistency)

rectal wall, empty or filled with feces

base of the bladder..

then remove your finger & see if there is any gush of gas or any blood on your finger..

At the end: cover the patient & thank him..

3- SURGERY   MEDICAL SKILL LAB..

Nasogastric tube placement:

First: greet the patient,

introduce yourself,

take permission,

hand washing,

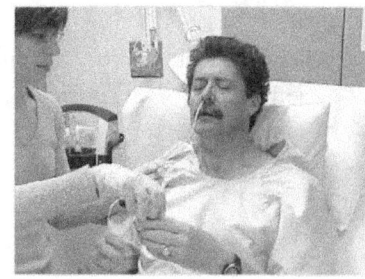

Make sure there is no trauma or any difficulty in breathing..

Check for obstruction, polyp or deviation..

Then measure the nasogastric tube length & mark it..
   (from the nose to the ear to the xiyphoid of sternum)

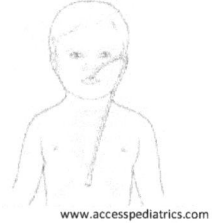

Then: wear a glove, put lubricant & introduce the tube..

  be carful that the tip of the tube must be pointed downward..

  When it reaches the **nasopharynx** (you will feel some kind of resistance).. So, you have to:

  twist the tube about 180°,

  ask the patient to drink water..

  & ***continue*** till you reach the marked point..

Everything is O.K. ??: make sure you are at a right place by one of the following:

   - push air by a syringe & auscultate for gastric bubble
   - by X-ray..
   - or can send an aspiration to the lab → gastric content..

At the end: fix the tube by a plaster, connect the tube to a collecting bag & thank him..

3- SURGERY — MEDICAL SKILL LAB..

Foley's catheter insertion:

First: greet the patient,
introduce yourself,
take permission,
hand washing,

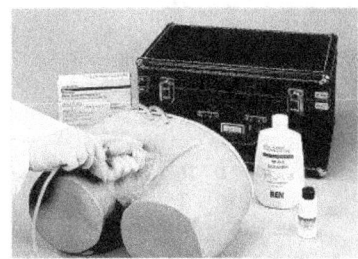

Make sure there is no trauma or bleeding from the external urethral meatus..

Wear gloves, lubricate the tip of the catheter & sterilize by povidone iodine (in circular manner) [in longitudinal manner in ♀ patients]

Then: in ♂ point the tip of the penis toward the ceiling [separate the labia majora in ♀],

put lidocaine by a syringe to the urethra and wait for 3-5 min.,

ask the patient to take a shallow breath and gently insert the catheter,

fill the balloon by 10 cc. of normal saline or air by a syringe,

then try to pull the catheter to make sure the right position of the catheter

At the end: connect the tube to a collecting bag, fix the tube by a plaster & thank him..

How to remove Foley's catheter:

wear a glove,
empty the balloon by a syringe,
gently try to pull the catheter..

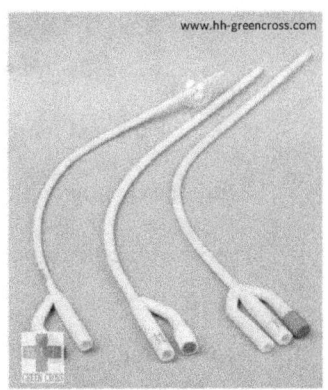

2 & 3 way Foley's catheters..

3- SURGERY MEDICAL SKILL LAB..

Cannula insertion:

First: greet the patient,

introduce yourself,

take permission,

hand washing, wear gloves..

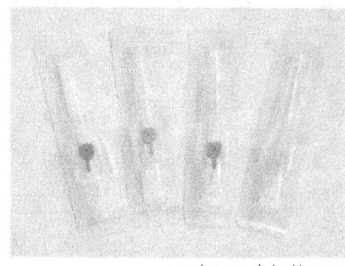
www.image.made-in-china.com

Then: Choose the size of the cannula you shall use. In general the larger gauge needle you use, the higher the maximum flow rate of the fluid entering into the vein.

Apply the tourniquet around the patient's arm and tighten appropriately.

Clean the skin using an alcohol wipe (in circular manner)

Insert the cannula at approximately 30 degrees.

Advance the cannula until a flashback is seen at the base (a flashback occurs when blood enters the base of the cannula).

The needle should now be held stationary whilst the plastic component of the cannula is advanced further into the vein.

Keep advancing the plastic component of the cannula until the plastic tube is fully inserted.

Remove the tourniquet from the patient's arm.

→ Trick: I do this step as soon as I see the flashback at the base.. to prevent any bleeding from the cannula.

Remove the needle from the base of the cannula leaving the plastic component in situ.

Take the bung and insert it into the end of the cannula.

Secure the cannula with an appropriate dressing.

Dispose of the sharps safely and any other waste.

At the end: thank him..

Chest tube placement:

First: greet the patient,

introduce yourself,

take permission,

hand washing, wear gloves

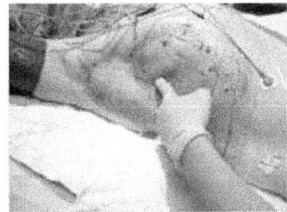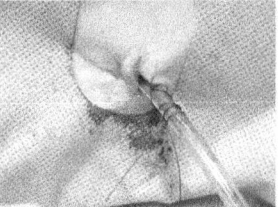

Site: Insertion should be in the ' *safe triangle* '. This is the triangle bordered by the anterior border of the latissimus dorsi, the lateral border of the pectoralis major muscle, a line superior to the horizontal level of the nipple, and an apex below the axilla.

Or roughly, 4th -5th intercostals space (at mid-axillary line) in hemothorax or
2nd intercostals space (at mid-clavicular line) in pneumothorax

Antiseptic: sterilize the insertion area.

Anesthesia: inject xylocaine by a syringe & wait 5 min.

The steps in insertion of a chest drain are as follows:

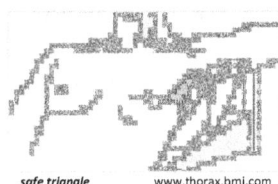

safe triangle www.thorax.bmj.com

- An incision (1 cm) is made along the upper border of the rib below the intercostal space to be used.
- The drain track will be directed over the top of the lower rib to avoid the intercostal vessels lying below each rib.
- The incision should easily accommodate the operator's finger.
- Using a curved clamp the track is developed by blunt dissection only. The clamp is inserted into muscle tissue and spread to split the fibres. The track is developed with the operator's finger.
- Once the track comes onto the rib, the clamp is angled just over the rib and dissection continued until the pleural is entered.
- A finger is inserted into the pleural cavity and the area explored for pleural adhesions. At this time the lung, diaphragm and heart may be felt..
- A large-bore (32 or 36F) chest tube is mounted on the clamp and passed along the track into the pleural cavity.
- The tube is connected to an underwater seal and sutured / secured in place.
- If desired, a U-stitch (or *purse string* suture) is placed for subsequent drain removal
- The chest is re-examined to confirm effect.
- A chest X-ray is taken to confirm placement & position.

At the end: thank him..

Purse string suture

3- SURGERY — MEDICAL SKILL LAB..

I.M. injection:

First: greet the patient,

introduce yourself,

take permission,

hand washing

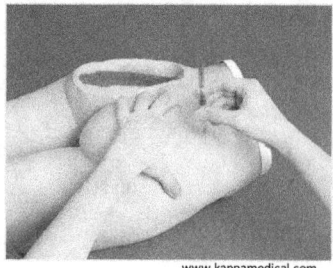

Then: **Drawing Up The Medicine Into The Syringe**

Selecting The Site For Injection: *' Buttock (Gluteus Medius) Site For I.M. Injection '*

- Find the trochanter. *It is the knobby top portion of the long bone in your upper leg (femur). It is the size of a golf ball.*
- Find the posterior iliac crest.
- Draw an imaginary line between the two bones.
- After locating the center of the imaginary line, find a point one inch toward your head. This is where (X) you will put the needle in.

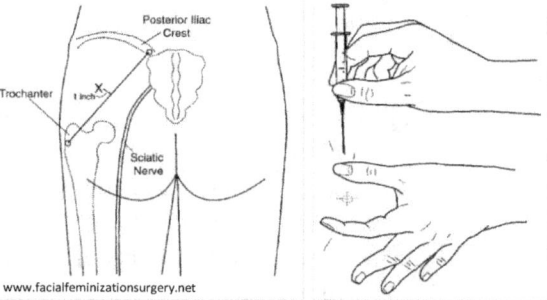

Giving The IM Injection

- Clean your skin with an alcohol pad in a circular motion. Let the alcohol dry. *Remove the needle cap and hold the syringe like a dart or pencil.*
- Stretch the skin at the injection site. *If you are thin, you may need to bunch the muscle up.*
- Insert the needle straight into the skin at a 90 degree angle. *Use a dart-like motion. Let go of the skin. Hold onto the syringe so that it will not move. Pull back on the plunger to make sure there is no blood. Remove the needle if you see blood in the syringe.*
- Inject the medicine by pushing down on the plunger at a moderate rate. *Be sure to inject all the medicine in the syringe. Remove the needle and quickly press the alcohol pad onto the site. Hold the pad tightly for a minute or until any bleeding stops. Check the area for any redness, bleeding or bruising.*

At the end: Put the used syringe and needle into a heavy plastic container and secure the cap.

Thank him..

3- SURGERY — MEDICAL SKILL LAB..

Indications, complications, contraindications & removal *'in brief'*:

NASOGASTRIC TUBE:

Indication: Acute intestinal obstruction
Acute peritonitis
Post op. in bowel surgery
Gastric hemorrhage
For feeding in comatose patient
To collect gastric lavage

Complication: Injury to the upper respiratory tract
Trauma to the pharynx or esophagus
Aspiration pneumonitis
Obstruction or kinking
Water & electrolyte imbalance
Dryness of the mouth

Indication of removal: There is normal bowel motion
No leak
No indication for it

FOLEY'S CATHETER:

Indication: Relive acute or chronic retention of urine or clot retntion
In all pelvic & perineal operations
Irrigation of urinary bladder
For measuring of urine output & urine sampling

Complication: Infection
Urethral injury
Urethral stricture

Contraindication: Local urethral sepsis
Urethral injury
Urethral stricture

I.V. CANNULA:

Indication: Taking blood sample
Giving blood or I.V. fluid
Giving drugs, injection of contrast medium
Parentral feeding

Complication: Bleeding or extravasation
Infection & Thrombophlebitis
Air embolism
Obstruction

3- SURGERY — MEDICAL SKILL LAB..

CHEST TUBE:

Indication: Pneumothorax
Hemothorax
pyothorax
chylothorax
Pleural effusion

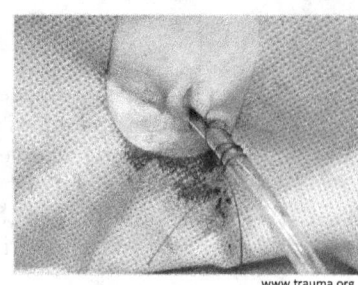

Complication: Allergic reaction
Trauma during insertion
Soft tissue bleeding
Infection
Obstruction, kinking or slipping of the drain

Indication of removal: Medical → the patient is well & normal breathing sounds
Mechanical → drain NOTHING..
By X-ray → full expansion of the lung

3- SURGERY — RADIOLOGY..

How to report ' THE CHEST X-RAY ':

First: This is a *plain* chest x-ray,

Posteroanterior view (or lateral view),

Taking for *Layla Rami, 25 y. old,
at the 2nd of October 2012,*

There is No rotation, good exposure,
with complete expiration

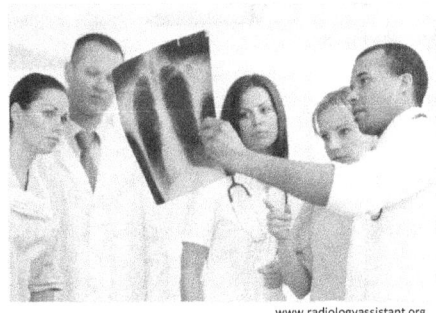

Showing: *' check for any abnormality in.. '*

Trachea,

Hilum,

Mediastinum (*measure it to see if there is any widening*),

Diaphragm & under diaphragm,

Heart (*measure it to see if there is any cardiomegaly*),

Hidden areas : *upper lung zone (apex)
costophrenic & cardiophrenic angles
retrocardiac..*

Lung,

Soft tissue & bones (shoulder, clavicle, ribs, vertebrae),

At the end: thank him..

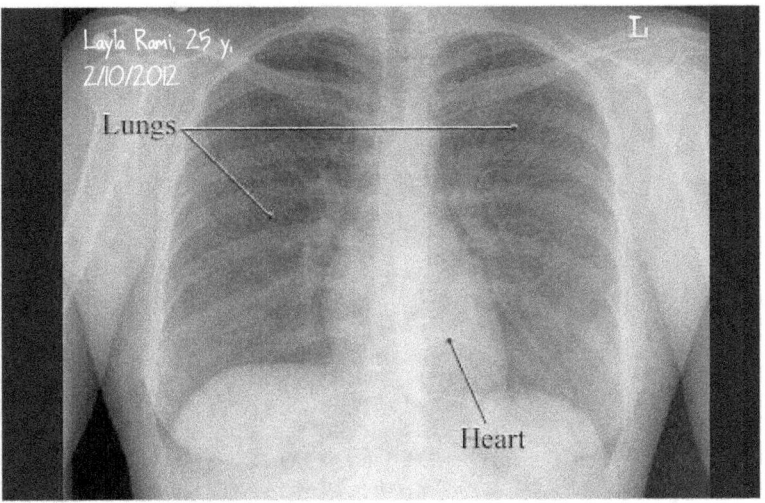

3- SURGERY — RADILOGY..

How to report ' THE ABDOMINAL X-RAY ':

First: This is a *plain* (*or contrast like swallow or Barium enema ..etc*) abdominal x-ray..

Posteroanterior view (*or lateral view*),

Taking for *Fatima Rami, 55 y. old, at the 10th of October 2012,*

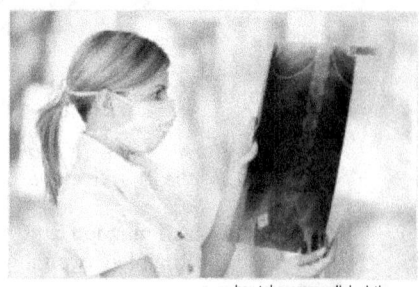

Showing: *' check for any abnormality in.. '*

Soft tissue (Liver, Spleen, Kidneys, Psoas muscles, ureters, bladder, uterus),

Gas shadow.. (*normal in stomach, 1st part of duodenum & large bowel*),

Air fluid levels,

Calcification,

At the end: thank him..

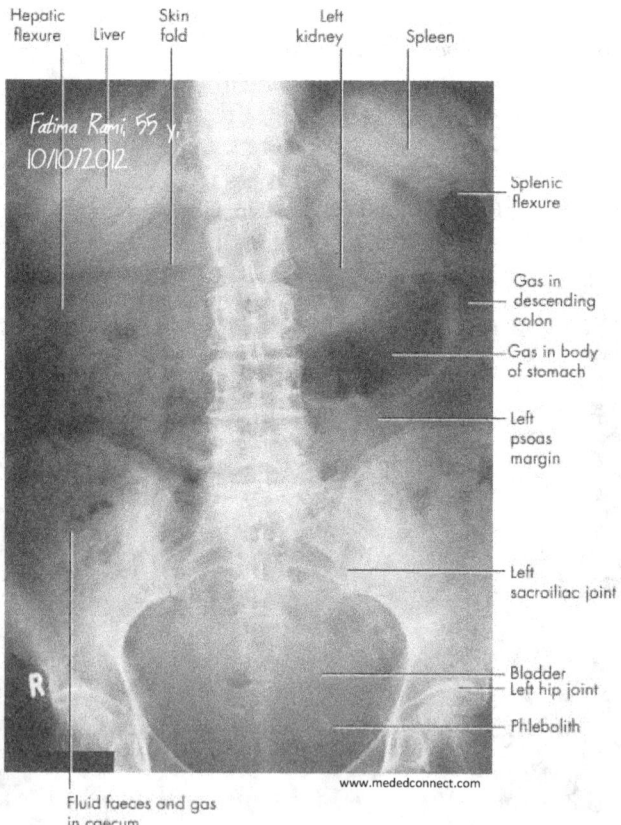

3- SURGERY — RADILOGY..

Some of important X-rays & Other radiological studies:

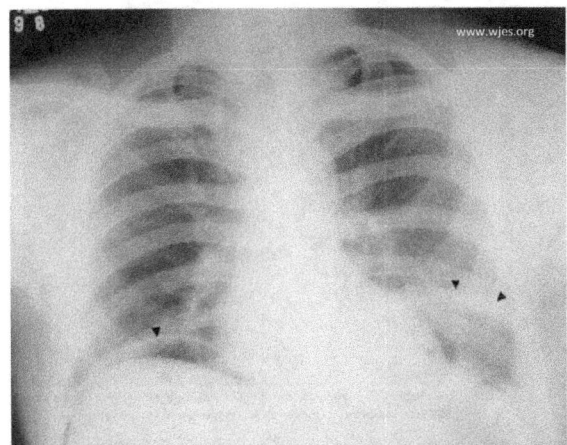
Air under diaphragm

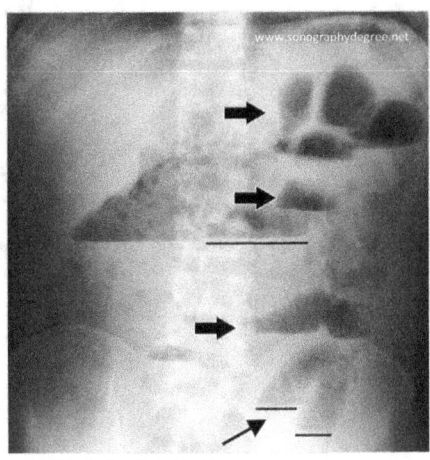
Air fluid levels - intestinal obstruction

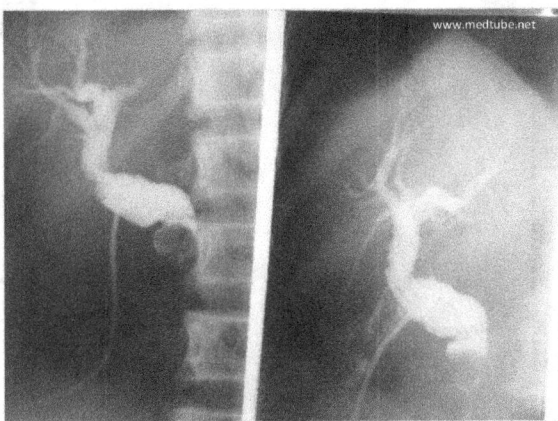
T-tube cholangiography show missed stone in the common bile duct

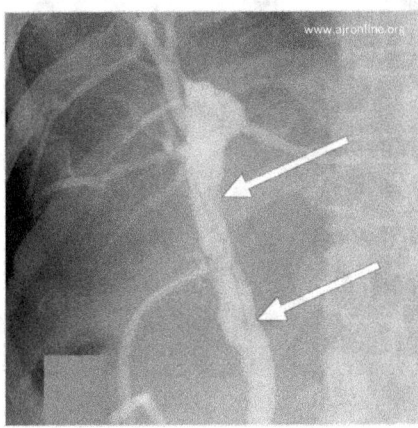
T-tube cholangiography image after cholecystectomy shows smooth indentation of bile duct (arrows).

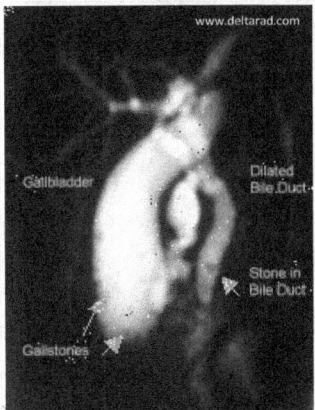
MRCP..

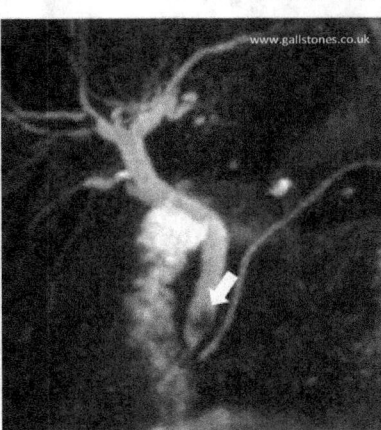
MRCP showing a stone in the lower bile duct.

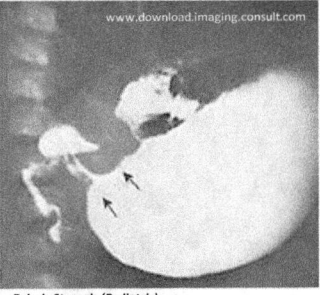
Pyloric Stenosis (Pediatric).

3- SURGERY   RADIOLOGY..

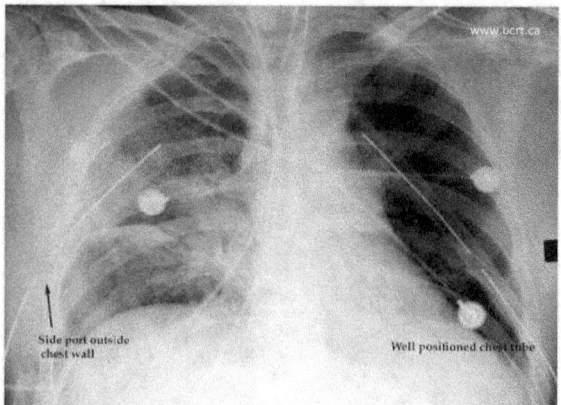

X-ray chest tube port outside..

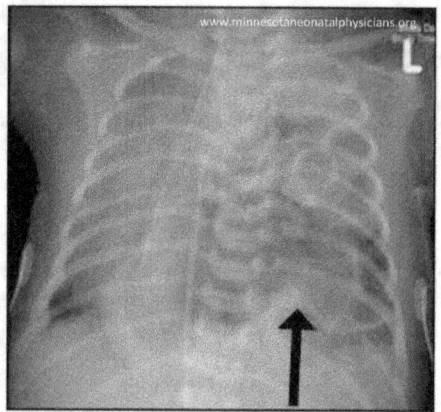

Congenital Diaphragmatic Hernia - Chest X-ray of patient with left-sided CDH. Arrow points to the stomach and intestine in the left chest cavity.

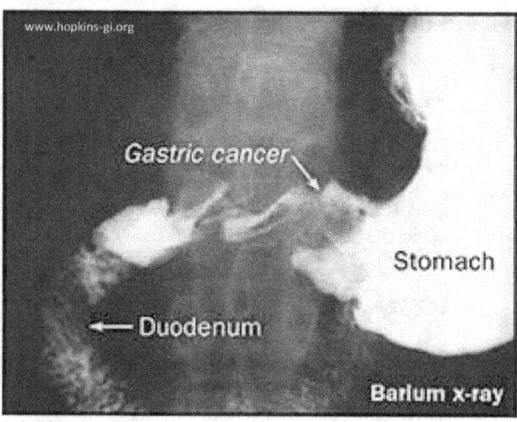

Gastric ca.

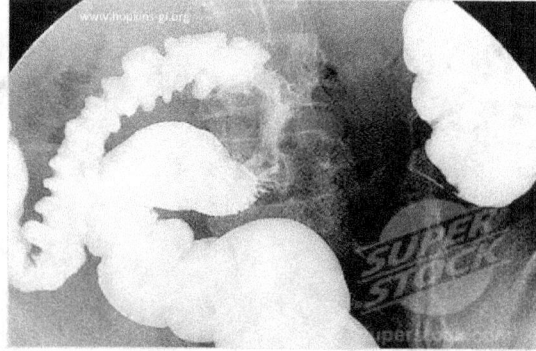

Colon cancer

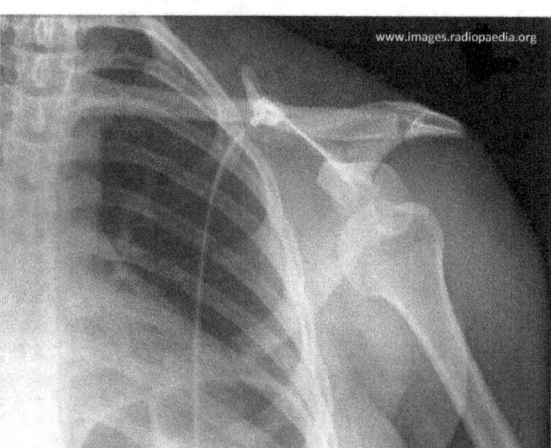

Anterior shoulder dislocation

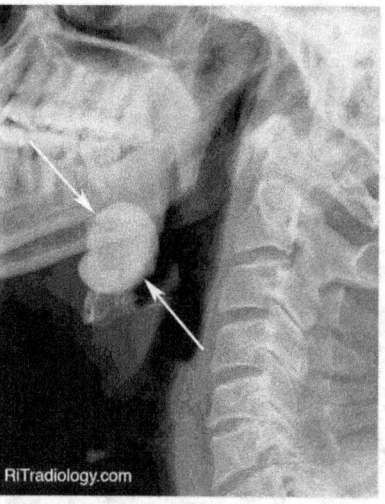

Sialolithiasis - Lateral radiograph of the neck shows a very large, well-defined calcification with layered appearance overlying the inferior aspect of the mandible.

3- SURGERY — UROSURGERY ' focus HISTORY TAKING '..

Genitourinary problems ' history taking ':

START WITH DEMOGRAPHY:

name, age, sex, marital state, address, occupation, date of admission & date of taking H_x,

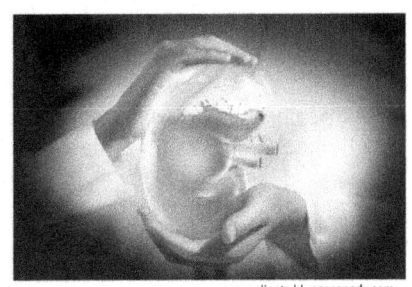

CHIEF COMPLAINT & DURATION:

H_x OF PRESENT ILLNESS:

You have to ask about.. *pain & hematuria*
Irritative & obstructive symptoms
Incontinence, retention & urgency

Urine (polyuria, oliguria, oder, ..etc)
Fever, discharge..etc

PAST MEDICAL H_x:
PAST SURGICAL H_x:
DRUG H_x:

Trick: Don't forget the H_x must be in the patient words.. So, instead of Oliguria → we say decrease in urine amount & so on..

FAMILY H_x:
SOCIOECONOMIC H_x:

SEXUAL H_x:

& don't forget the REVIEW of SYSTEMS:

IRRITATIVE SYMPTOMS:
- *Frequency*
- *Nacturia*
- *Dysuria*

OBSTRUCTIVE SYMPTOMS:
- *Hesitancy*
- *Straining*
- *↓↓ force of urination*
- *Intermittency*
- *Dribbling*

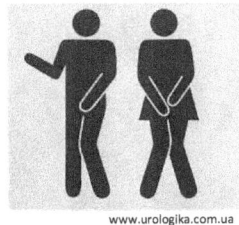

3- SURGERY — UROSURGERY ' focus HISTORY TAKING '..

Hematuria ' history taking ':

START WITH DEMOGRAPHY:

name, age, sex, marital state, address, occupation, date of admission & date of taking Hx,

CHIEF COMPLAINT & DURATION:

Hx OF PRESENT ILLNESS:

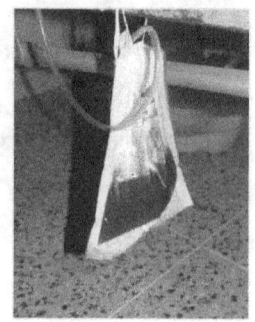

continuous or intermitted,
painful or painless,
any clots ? + shape of the clots..
in the beginning, end or total of the stream ?
irritative & other urological symptoms..

in ♀ patient.. the menstrual Hx is very important.

PAST MEDICAL Hx: bleeding tendency..
PAST SURGICAL Hx:
DRUG Hx:

FAMILY Hx:
SOCIOECONOMIC Hx: smoker ?, food or beverages ingestion ?

& don't forget the REVIEW of SYSTEMS:

Pain ' history taking ':

It is similar as any branch in medicine or surgery..

Described previously.. see page 62 ..

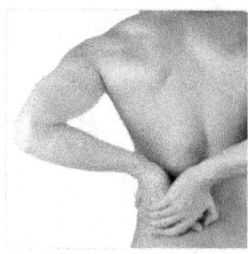

3- SURGERY — UROSURGERY ' EXAMINATION '..

Abdominal examination:

Described previously in details *in chapter ' 1 '..*
See page 23 ..

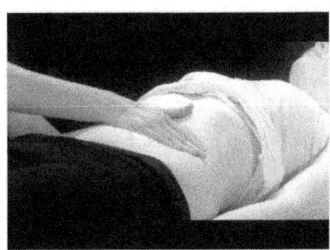

In *UROSURGERY* you have to concentrate on the following:

- Bimanual palpation of the kidneys & *renal angle tenderness* (*from the back*)
- Palpation & percussion of the bladder
- Auscultation of the renal bruit

- *At the end*, mention the genitalia & P.R examination..

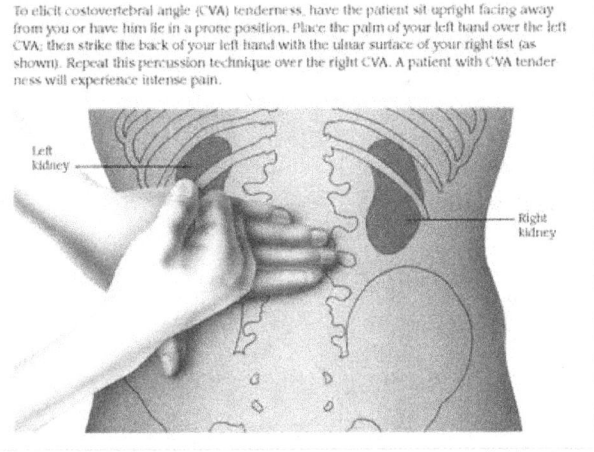

EXAMINATION TIP
Eliciting CVA tenderness

To elicit costovertebral angle (CVA) tenderness, have the patient sit upright facing away from you or have him lie in a prone position. Place the palm of your left hand over the left CVA; then strike the back of your left hand with the ulnar surface of your right fist (as shown). Repeat this percussion technique over the right CVA. A patient with CVA tenderness will experience intense pain.

3- SURGERY — UROSURGERY ' EXAMINATION '..

General Examination related to urosurgery:

General look: pallor, tired, in pain, breathlessness, hydration, bruising & itching marks..

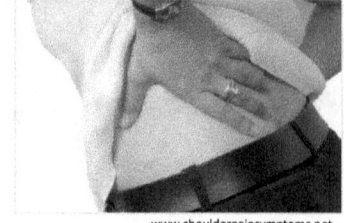

Hand: leukonychia, koilonychias, half & half nails,

flapping tremor,

radial pulse & B.P.

Face: plethoric face (earthy color)

pallor (or jaundice ??)

Lung: crackles ??..

Then do complete Abdominal examination..

Leg: edema & peripheral neuropathy

3- SURGERY — UROSURGERY 'EXAMINATION'..

Genital examination:

First: greet the patient,

introduce yourself,

take permission for examination,

hand washing,

make sure patient privacy,

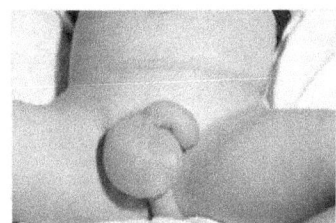

good exposure *' Genital area & upper thigh '* **& you need** *gloves..*

Inspection: any redness, swelling, ulcer, scar, incision & hair distribution

- Ask the patient to *cough* (Hernia ??)

- **Penis** → size, shape, color of skin, foreskin (circumcised ??.. *if not retract it*), external urethral meatus (E.U.M.) position,

- **Scrotum** → skin (well developed or not ?), symmetry, discoloration, discharge, don't forget to examine the back of the scrotum..

Palpation: *ask the patient if he has any pain..*

- temperature, tenderness

- **Penis** → try to retract the foreskin & try to press around the E.U.M. to open it..

- **Scrotum** → testis (*size, consistency & any mass*)

Epididymis & spermatic cord..

If you can't palpate the testis.. you have to palpate the groin (may be undescended testis or retractile testis)..

If there is any *mass* you have to describe it as mentioned before (especially the transillumination).   see page 72 ..

L.N. & mention the P.R. and abdominal examination..

At the end: cover the patient, thank him..

3- SURGERY — UROSURGERY ' RADIOLOGY '..

How to report ' UROSURGERY - RADIOLOGICAL STUDIES ':

PLAIN & CONTRAST X-RAY:

First: This is a *plain (K.U.B.)* or *contrast(I.V.U)* or *contrast voiding X-ray..*

Taking for *Fatima Rami, 55 y. old, at the 10th of October 2012,*
30 min. after contrast administration..

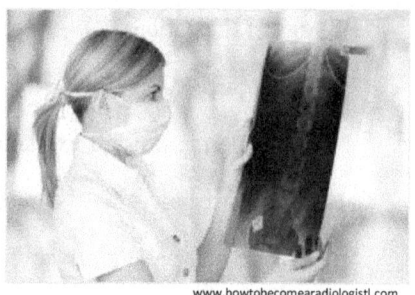

Showing: ' *check for any abnormality in..* '

Both kidneys, ureters, part of the pelvis, vertebrae & bladder,
Good quality,
Normal kidneys parenchymal shadow,
Normal psoas muscles margin shadows..

In **K.U.B** → any radio-opaque stone (staghorn stone ?), parenchymal humb,
bladder stone..
calcification or gases or *Double J stent*
mal-rotated kidney

In **I.V.U.** → Calyces (*cupped = normal*) or (*clubbed = abnormal*)
Dilated pelvis (hydronephrosis)
Filling defect in the pelvis

Dilated ureter (hydroureter)
Stricture

Bladder abnormality

In **voiding** → any reflux.. (you can see a *tube* through the urethra)..

At the end: thank the patient..

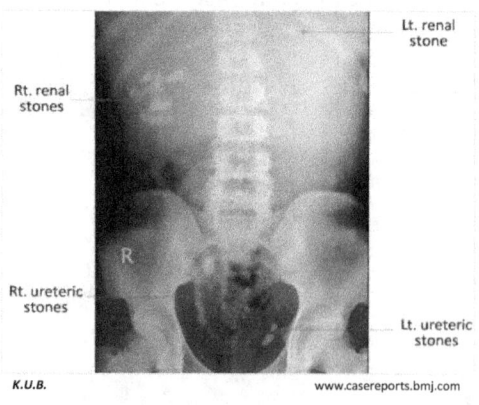
K.U.B. www.casereports.bmj.com

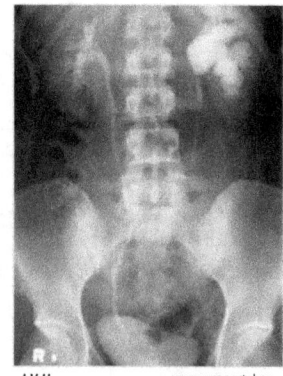
I.V.U. www.uroportal.ru

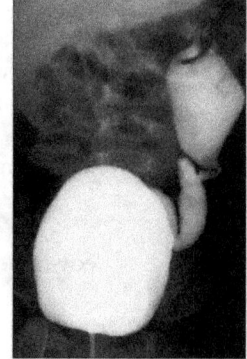
Contrast voiding x-ray www.ajronline.org

3- SURGERY — UROSURGERY ' RADIOLOGY '..

CT SCAN:

First: This is a *CT scan (native or contrast)*, taking for *Fatima Rami, 55 y. old, at the 10ᵗʰ of October 2012*,

Showing: ' check for any abnormality in.. '

In native..
The lower part of the abdomen & pelvic region (*you can know that from the K.U.B. placed in the left upper corner of every CT scan*),
Any stone in the kidneys (*stoghorn stone ?*), ureters or bladder..

In contrast..
Hydronephrosis,
Functioning kidneys ??
Parenchymal lesions (*enhanced → may be Ca., not enhanced → may be cyst*)

Trick: You can recognize many of abnormalities by comparing between the two kidneys & ureters..

At the end: thank him..

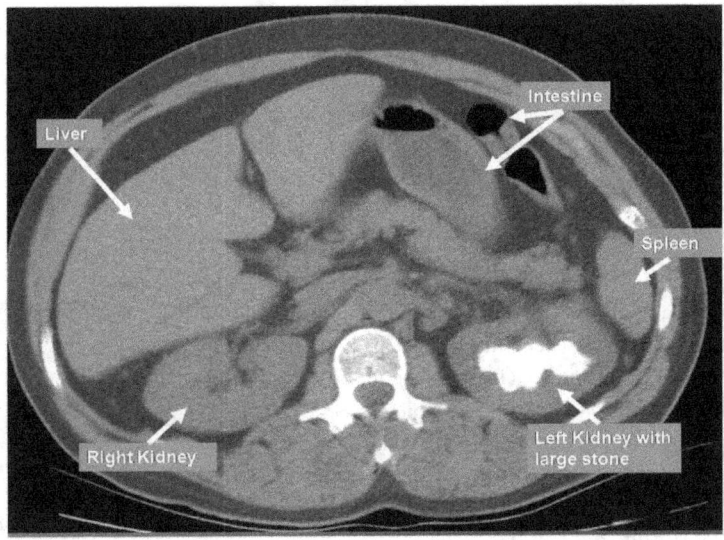

CT scan

3- SURGERY

UROSURGERY 'INSTRUMENTS'..

UROSURGERY - INSTRUMENTS:

DOUBLE J STENT:

A double J stent is a soft tube that is placed during surgery. This tube has a curl at both ends designed to prevent the stent from moving down into the bladder or up into the kidney.

Some stents have a string attached to them which exits from the urethra. Stents are placed in the ureter.

A stent is placed to prevent or relieve a blockage in the ureter. After many stone surgeries the small pieces of stone can drop down into the ureter and block it, causing severe pain and occasionally infection. A stent allows the ureter to dilate, which makes it easier for stones or stone fragments to pass.

Other surgeries in which stents are used includes:
- Removal of tumors from either the ureter or the kidney
- Repair of scars in the ureter
- Removal of tumors from around the ureter

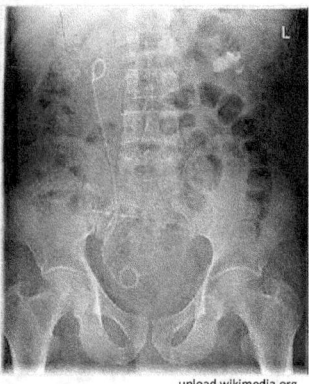
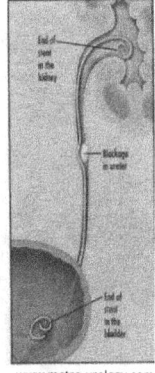

CYSTOSCOPE:

Cystoscopy may be recommended for any of the following conditions:

- Urinary tract infections
- Blood in the urine (hematuria)
- Loss of bladder control (incontinence) or overactive bladder
- Unusual cells found in urine sample
- Need for a bladder catheter
- Painful urination, chronic pelvic pain, or interstitial cystitis
- Urinary blockage such as from prostate enlargement, stricture, or narrowing of the urinary tract
- Stone in the urinary tract
- Unusual growth, polyp, tumor, or cancer

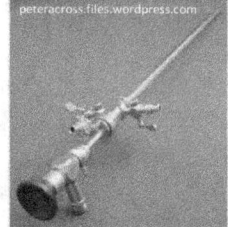
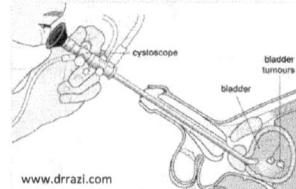

CHAPTER 4

ORTHOPEDICS

Contents:

EXAMINATION	
Shoulder joint	112
Elbow joint	114
Hip joint	116
Knee joint	118
Wrist & hand	120
Ankle joint & foot	122
Back (Lumbar spine)	124
Neck (Cervical spine)	126
HOW TO REPORT ' The orthopedics & fracture X-ray '	128

4- ORTHOPEDIC EXAMINATION..

Shoulder joint examination:

First: greet the patient,

introduce yourself,

take permission for examination,

hand washing,

make sure patient privacy,

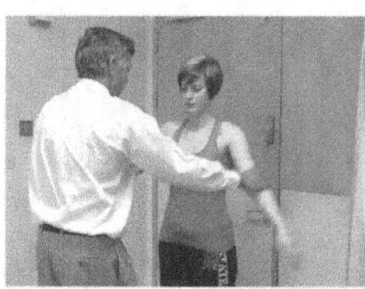

good exposure *' both shoulders, arms, chest & neck '*

Look: *(from anterior, lateral & posterior)*

symmetry, deformity, at the same levels ?, scapular outlines,

swelling or redness, wasting, scar, sinus,

push against the wall (for winging of scapula) → lesion of the serratus ant. m. $C_{5,6,7}$.

Feel: *' ask him if he has any pain '..*

temperature & tenderness (from sternoclavicular → acromioclavicular joint → acromion process → supraspinatus tenderness, long head of biceps.. edge of the scapula)

Move: **active..** forward flexion (0-170°), extension (0-40°),
abduction (0-160° *'painful arc ?'*), adduction,
internal rotation (0-90°), external rotation (0-70°),
also scapula movement..

→ Trick: Observe the range, symmetry & rhythm of the movements..

then **passive..** *here, you have to feel the joint by the other hand to feel any crepitus..*

' during the examination you have to observe the biceps function & painful arc..'

Special tests: Apley scratch test & Apprehension test..

Don't forget: neurovascular examination → brachial a., axillary a. & subclavian a.
power, reflexes *' biceps & triceps '*,
sensation *' axillary n. '*

L.N. *' axillary & supraclavicular '*

Suggest to examine the proximal & distal joints..

At the end: cover the patient, thank him..

4- ORTHOPEDIC EXAMINATION..

References: www.osceskills.com
Apley's System of Orthopaedics and Fractures

Some of helpful images for ' shoulder examination ':

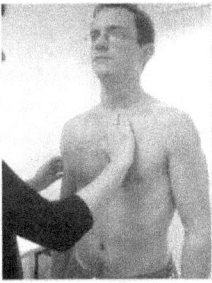
Sternoclavicular - joint palpation

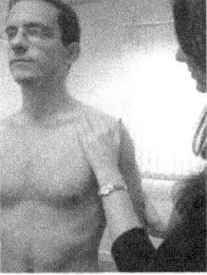
Acromioclavicular - joint palpation

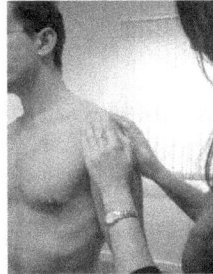
Glenohumeral - joint palpation

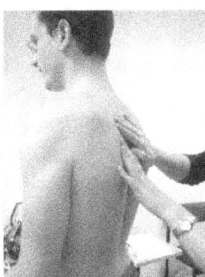
Spine of the scapula - joint palpation

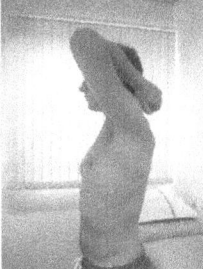
Flexion - movement

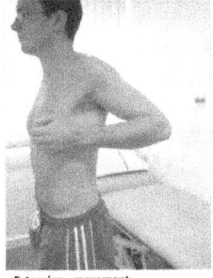
Extension - movement

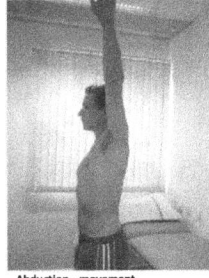
Abduction - movement

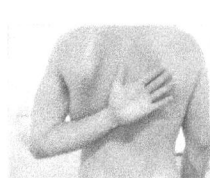
Internal rotation - movement

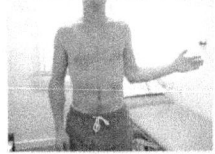
External rotation - movement

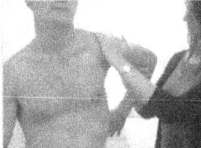
Impingement test

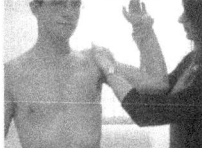
Apprehension test

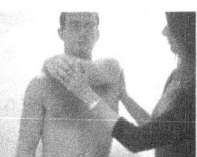
Scarf test

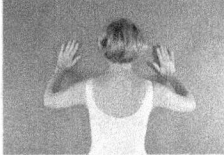
Testing for serratus anterior weakness

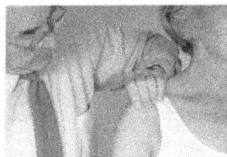
Feeling for supraspinatus tenderness.

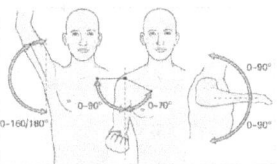
Normal range of movement

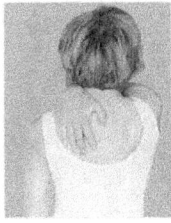
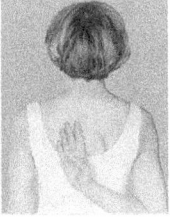
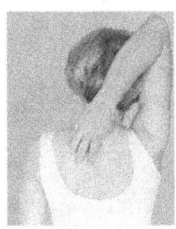

Scratch test: 'Shoulder' pain may be due to disorders of the shoulder joint itself (e.g. gleno-humeral arthritis), the acromioclavicular joint (injury or arthritis) or structures around the joint (e.g. the rotator cuff syndromes). But it could also be referred from more distant lesions (e.g. brachial neuralgia, cervical spondylosis or cardiac ischaemia). If the patient can scratch the opposite scapula in these three ways, the shoulder joint and its tendons are unlikely to be at fault.

4- ORTHOPEDIC EXAMINATION..

Elbow joint examination:

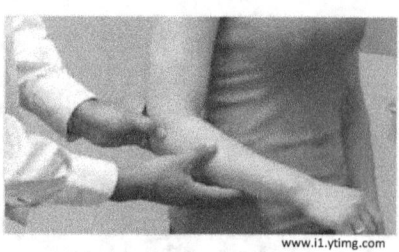

First: greet the patient,
introduce yourself,
take permission for examination,
hand washing,
make sure patient privacy,
good exposure

Look: *(from anterior, lateral & posterior)*

symmetry, deformity, at the same levels ?, *carrying angle 5-10°*,

swelling or redness, wasting, scar, sinus,

olecranon bursa..

Feel: ' *ask him if he has any pain* '..
temperature & tenderness (medial & lateral epicondyles + olecranon process)

*lateral epicondyle → Tennis elbow ' intensified by active extension of the wrist ',
medial epicondyle → Golfer elbow,*

palpate & tap on the ulner n.

Move: **active..** full extension (0°), full flexion (140°),
pronation (90°), supination (90°),
internal rotation (0-90°), external rotation (0-70°),
also scapula movement..

then **passive..** *here, you have to feel the joint by the other hand to feel any crepitus..*

Special tests: Tennis & Golfer elbow (done with palpation)..

Don't forget: neurovascular examination → brachial a. & radial a.,
power, reflexes,
sensation..

L.N. ' *epitrochlear* '
Suggest to examine the proximal & distal joints..

At the end: cover the patient, thank him..

4- ORTHOPEDIC EXAMINATION..

References: www.osceskills.com
Apley's System of Orthopaedics and Fractures

Some of helpful images for ' Elbow examination ':

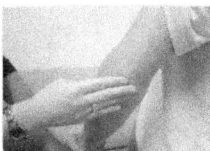
Palpate the olecranon process

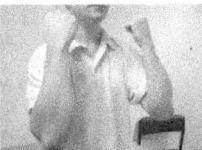
Flexion-movement

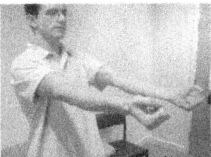
Extension-movement

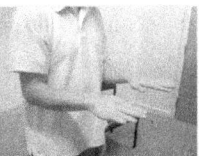
Pronation-movement

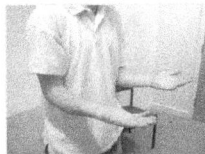
Supination-movement

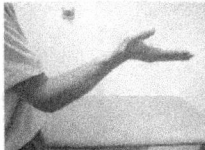
Tennis-elbow-assessment

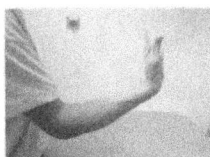
Golfers-elbow-assessment

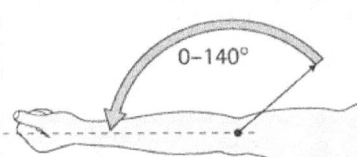
Normal range of movement

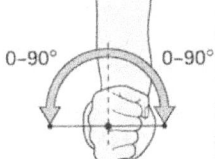
Tennis elbow - Pain provoked by resisted wrist extension

4- ORTHOPEDIC EXAMINATION..

Hip joint examination:

Must be in 3 positions:
Supine, sitting & lying position..

First: greet the patient,
introduce yourself,
take permission for examination,
hand washing,
make sure patient privacy,
good exposure ' when needed.. '

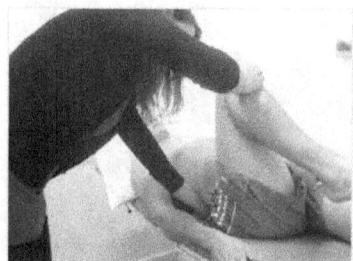

Then: Trendelenburg's test,
Gait,
Iliopsoas function (in sitting positions)..

→ Trick: It is worth to start by special tests in hip examination

Look: symmetry (both A.S.I.S at same level), deformity,
swelling or redness, wasting, scar, sinus,
legs length → 2 methods → (Aapparent: from Xiphisternum to medial malleolus)
(Real: from A.S.I.S. to malleolus)

Feel: ' ask him if he has any pain '..
temperature & tenderness (ischial tuberosity, greater trochanter & tendon of adductor longus)

Move: ' you have to support the pelvis by one hand to prevent its movement '..
active.. flexion (0-140°) → *THOMAS test* ,
abduction (0-40°), adduction (0-20°),
internal rotation (0-50°), external rotation (0-30°),
then **passive..**

Special tests: done in previous steps..

Then: prone position (from the back) → *scar, swelling, sinus, wasting ' glutei & hamstring m. ', tuft of hair, tenderness & extension (0-10°)..*

Don't forget: neurovascular examination & L.N. examination (inguinal)..
Suggest to examine the proximal & distal joints..

At the end: cover the patient, thank him..

4- ORTHOPEDIC EXAMINATION..

** References: www.osceskills.com
Apley's System of Orthopaedics and Fractures

Some of helpful images for ' Hip examination '.

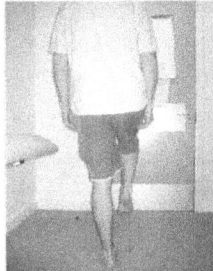
Trendelenberg test

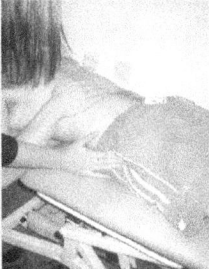
Palpation of the greater trochanter

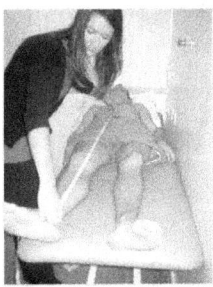
Apparent length assessment

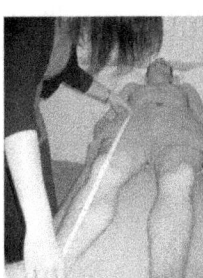
True length assessment

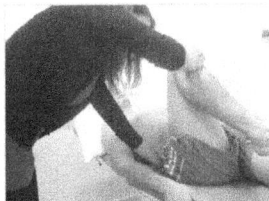
Place your hand under the patient's lumbar spine to stop any lumbar movements and fully flex one of the hips. Observe the other hip, if it lifts off the couch then it suggests a fixed flexion deformity of that hip.

Thomas test

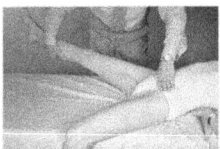
Abduction - movement

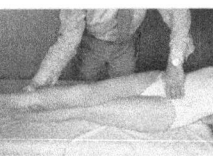
Adduction - movement

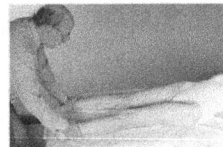
External & internal rotation - movement

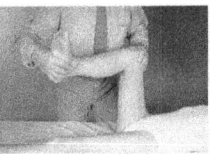
Internal rotation in 90° of hip flexion - movement

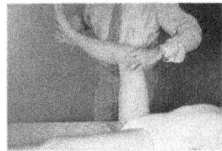
External rotation in 90° of hip flexion - movement

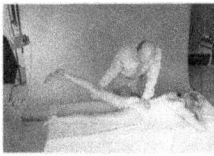
Extension - movement

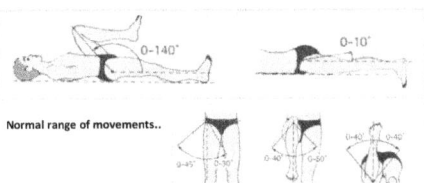
Normal range of movements..

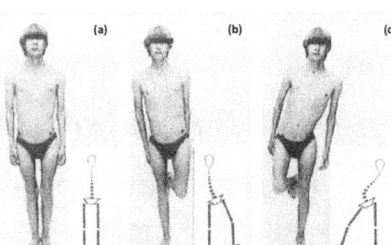

Trendelenburg's sign (a) Standing normally on two legs. **(b)** tanding on the right leg which has a normal hip whose bductor muscles ensure correct weight transference. **(c)** Standing on the left leg whose hip is faulty, and so abduction cannot be achieved; the pelvis drops on the unsupported side and the shoulder swings over to the left.

4- ORTHOPEDIC EXAMINATION..

Knee joint examination:

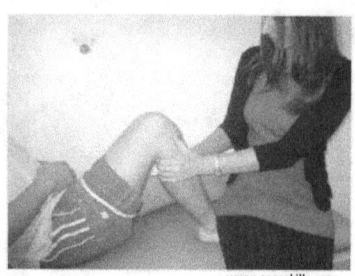

First: greet the patient,
introduce yourself,
take permission for examination,
hand washing,
make sure patient privacy,
good exposure *' when needed.. '*

Then: Gait,

Look: *symmetry,* deformity, swelling or redness, wasting, scar, sinus,
shape, position & symmetry of the **patella**

Feel: *' ask him if he has any pain '..*
temperature & tenderness (joint line, ligaments attachment, patella, patellar ligament)
asses joint effusion → patellar taping & milking
posterior surface of the patella

Move: **active..** flexion, extension,
rotation (the knee must be bent) → McMurray's test → may feel clunk..

then **passive..**

Special tests: valgus & varus stress tests,
Drawer tests (anterior & posterior)
Lachman test
Crude test
Patellar apprehension test
Sag sign

Then: prone position (from the back) → scar, swelling, Baker's cyst, aneurysm,
Grinding test & Destruction test

Don't forget: neurovascular examination & L.N. examination (popliteal)..
Suggest to examine the proximal & distal joints..

At the end: cover the patient, thank him..

4- ORTHOPEDIC EXAMINATION..

** References: www.osceskills.com
Apley's System of Orthopaedics and Fractures

Some of helpful images for ' Knee examination ':

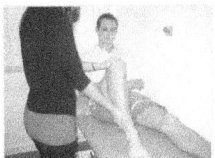 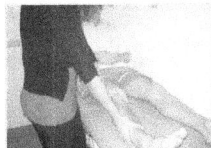 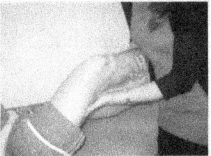 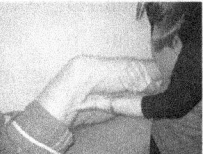

Flexion - movement   Extension - movement   Lateral and medial stress - internal   Latera and medial stress - external

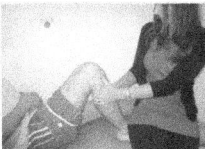

Drawer tests

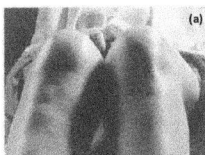 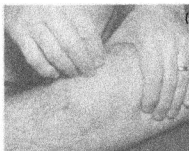 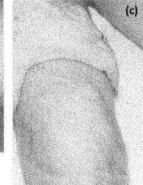 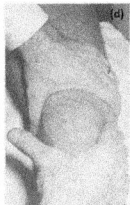 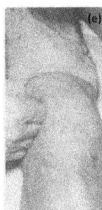

Testing for intra-articular fluid (a) The juxtapatellar hollow, which disappears in flexion if there is fluid in the knee. **(b)** Patellar tap test. **(c,d,e) Doing the bulge test:** compress the suprapatellar pouch *(c)*, empty the medial compartment *(d)*, push fluid back from the lateral compartment and watch for the bulge on the medial side *(e)*.

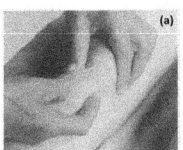 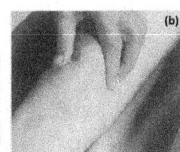

Patello-femoral joint:
(a) Feeling under the edge of the patella.
(b) Testing for patellofemoral tenderness.
(c) The patellar apprehension test

4- ORTHOPEDIC EXAMINATION..

Wrist & Hand examination:

First: greet the patient,
introduce yourself,
take permission for examination,
hand washing,
make sure patient privacy,
good exposure *'when needed..'*
you can ask about the hand dominance..

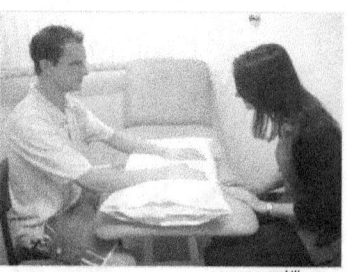

Look: *symmetry,* deformity, swelling or redness, wasting, scar, sinus,
skin (smooth, moist, dry & contracture..etc), callosities (working man's hand),
palmar creases (pallor), plamar erythema..
nails → pitting or other changes
(examine the palmar, dorsal surface of the hand & even the extensor surface of the forearm)..

Feel: *'ask him if he has any pain '..*
temperature, nodules,
tenderness → (styloid process in De Quervain's Tendinitis), (snuffbox in scaphoid injury), (ulnar head in extensor carpi ulnaris tendinitis)..
some schools say ' you can use fingers squeeze..'
palpate for dupuytren's contracture, flexor sheaths & crepitus with movement..

don't forget neurovascular examination (capillary refilling, radial a., ulnar a. & taping on the ulnar n.)

Move: **active..** flexion (0-80°) *'reverse prayer sign '*, extension (0-80°) *' prayer sign '*,
ulnar deviation (0-40°), radial deviation (0-10°),
pronation & supination (the elbow joint must keep stable),
thumb movments..

(**For more details,** you can see Chapter *1 – Nervous system examination*)

then **passive..**

Special tests: Finkelstein test (for De Quervain's Tendinitis), phalen (for flexion) & reverse phalen tests → *all done with palpation..*

Don't forget: neurovascular examination (*Allen's test is included..*), L.N. examination & function of hand assessment..
Suggest to examine the proximal joints..

At the end: cover the patient, thank him..

4- ORTHOPEDIC EXAMINATION..

** References: www.osceskills.com
Apley's System of Orthopaedics and Fractures

Some of helpful images for *Wrist & Hand examination*:

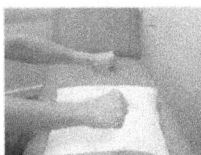
Finger flexion - movement

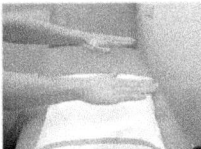
Finger extension - movement

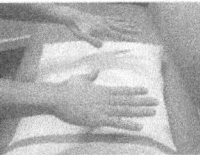
Finger abduction - movement

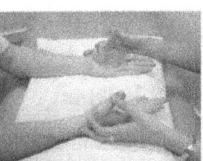
Finger abduction - movement

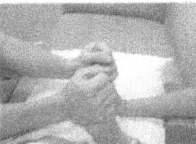
Power grip assessment

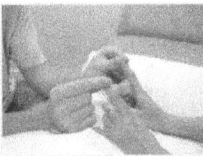
Pincer grip assessment

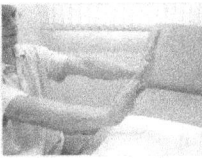
Wrist extension - movement

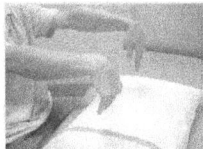
Wrist flexion - movement

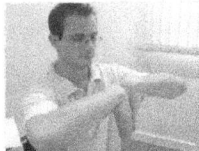
Phalens test

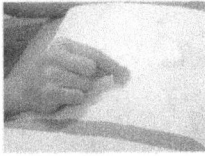
Pick up assessment

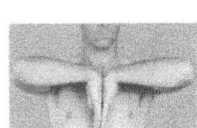
This is a good way to test flexion and extension of the wrists; you can compare the two sides.

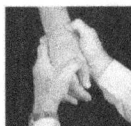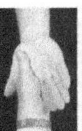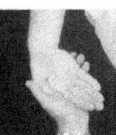
De Quervain's disease: (a) There is point tenderness at the tip of the radial styloid process. (b,c) Finkelstein's test:
Ulnar deviation with the thumb left free is relatively painless (b), but if the movement is repeated with the thumb held close to the palm (c), the pull on the thumb tendons causes intense pain.

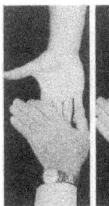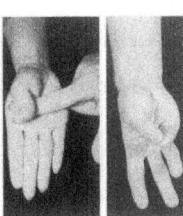
Thumb movements: You should have no difficulty defining the planes of movement if you follow this routine: (a) hold the patient's hand flat on the table and instruct him or her to 'stretch to the side' (extension), (b) 'point to the ceiling' (abduction), (c) 'pinch my finger' (adduction) and (d) 'touch your little finger' (opposition).

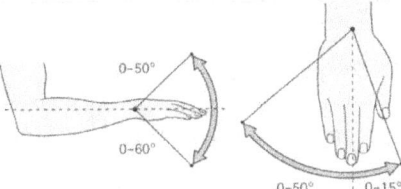
Normal range of movements

4- ORTHOPEDIC EXAMINATION..

Ankle joint & Foot examination:

Must be in 4 positions:
- the patient facing you,
- his back facing you,
- walking,
- tip toe walking..

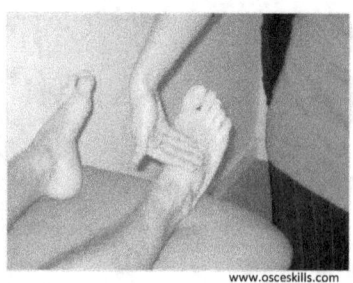

First: greet the patient,
introduce yourself,
take permission for examination,
hand washing,
make sure patient privacy,
good exposure *' when needed.. '*

Then: Gait,

Look: *symmetry,* deformity, swelling or redness, ulcer, wasting, scar, sinus,
observe the → Achilles tendon, heel, medial longitudinal arch, sole & nails..

Feel: *' ask him if he has any pain '..*
temperature & tenderness (joints, joint line, under medial arch → planter fasciitis, on the sesamoid bones → sesamoiditis, adjacent side of the 3rd & 4th toes → Morton's metatarsalgia),
some schools say ' you can use fingers squeeze..'

Move: **active..** dorsiflexion (0-15°), plantarflexion (0-40°),
inversion (0-30°), eversion,
toes movements → flexion & extension..

then **passive..**

Then: prone position (from the back) → *calf & ankle examination*

Special tests: Simmond' test → for Achilles tendon rupture..

Don't forget: neurovascular examination & L.N. examination (popliteal)..
Suggest to examine the proximal & distal joints..
See the shoes → may be medical one..

At the end: cover the patient, thank him..

4- ORTHOPEDIC EXAMINATION..

** References: www.osceskills.com
Apley's System of Orthopaedics and Fractures

Some of helpful images for ' Ankle joint & Foot examination ':

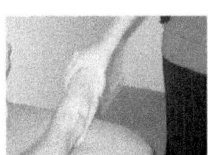
Squeeze over the metatarsophalangeal joints

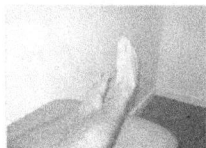
Inversion – movement - 1

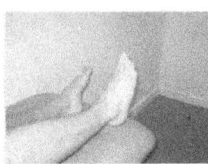
Inversion – movement - 2

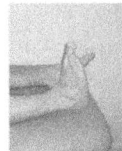
Eversion - movement t - 1

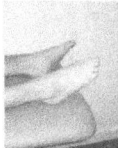
Eversion - movement - 2

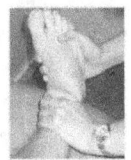
Passive inversion – movement

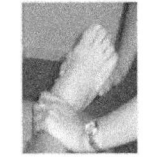
Passive eversion - movement

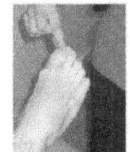
Toe plantarflexion - movement

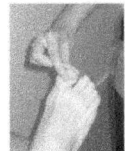
Toe dorsiflexion - movement

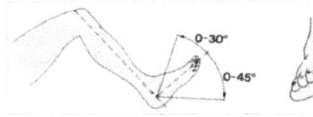
Normal range of movement

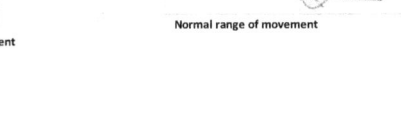

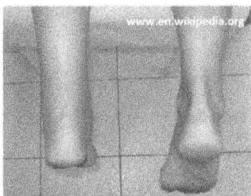
Simmonds' test: both calves are being squeezed but only the right foot plantarflexes – the left tendon is ruptured.

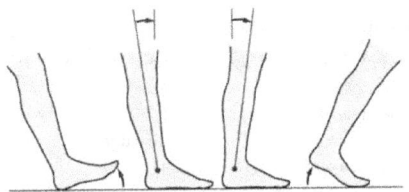
Gait – the three rockers of ankle-stance phase The first rocker begins with heel-strike – if the anterior compartment muscles are weak, a 'foot-slap' is noticeable; or if the ankle is in fixed equinus, this rocker may be absent altogether. In mid-stance, the centre of gravity of the body (and ground reaction force) moves from a position posterior to the ankle joint to anterior (second rocker). The third rocker produces an acceleration force that shifts the fulcrum of the pivot forwards to the metatarsal heads, just prior to toe-off (Gage, 1991).

4- ORTHOPEDIC EXAMINATION..

Back *(Lumbar spine)* examination:

Must be in 3 positions:
- upright,
- prone,
- supine position..

First: greet the patient,
introduce yourself,
take permission for examination,
hand washing & warming,
make sure patient privacy,
good exposure ' *both legs & the trunk should also be exposed* '

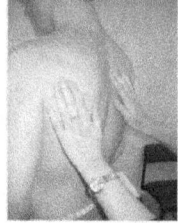

Look: *symmetry*, deformity, swelling or redness, hair tuft, wasting, scar, sinus,
skin lesion (café au lait, herpes zoster ..etc)

from the back → look again, hyperkyphosis, hyperlordosis, scoliosis or gibbus..
pelvis level

stand on his toes ($S_{1,2}$), heels ($L_{4,5}$), gaits..

Feel: ' *ask him if he has any pain* '..
temperature & spinous process for *tenderness & steps..*
finger breadth

Move: **active..** extension (lean forward), flexion,
lumber excursion → normally at least ↑↑ 5 cm.
lateral flexion (bend sideway) → 30°
rotation (you have to stabilize the pelvis) → 40°

Special tests: Femoral stretch test ($L_{2,3,4}$),
Siatic stretch test *(straight leg raising)* + passive dorsiflexion + confirmatory test,
FABER maneuver (for sacroiliac joint),
Heel – hip – occiput test (for ankylosing spondylitis)

Don't forget: neurovascular examination → hamstring power $L_{4,5}$, gluteus maximus power,
knee extension $L_{3,4}$, big toe dorsiflexion L_5, Planter flexion S_1, foot
inversion L_5 & eversion S_1..
then Reflexes, Sensation (saddle area $S_{3,4}$) & anal reflex $S_{4,5}$

L.N. examination.. abdomen for aortic aneurysm..
Suggest to examine the proximal & distal joints..

At the end: cover the patient, thank him..

4- ORTHOPEDIC EXAMINATION..

** References: www.osceskills.com
Apley's System of Orthopaedics and Fractures

Some of helpful images for ' Back (Lumbar spine) examination ':

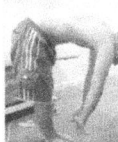 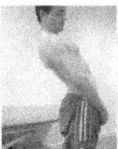 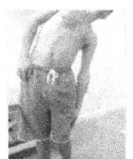 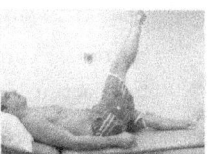

Flexion - movement   Extension - movement   Lateral flexion - movement   Straight leg raise..

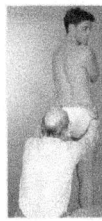

Hold the pelvis stable and ask the patient to twist first to one side and then to the other (rotation). Note that rotation occurs almost entirely in the thoracic spine and not in the lumbar spine.

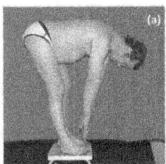 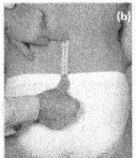 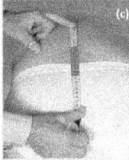

Measuring the range of flexion: Bending down and touching the toes may look like lumbar flexion but this is not always the case. The patient in (a) has ankylosing spondylitis and a rigid lumbar spine, but he is able to reach his toes because he has good flexibility at the hips. You can measure the lumbar excursion. With the patient upright, select two bony points 10 cm apart and mark the skin (b); as the patient bends forward, the two points should separate by at least a further 5 cm (c).

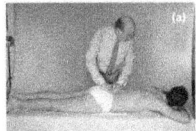 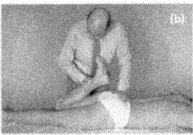 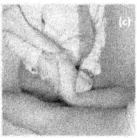

Examination with the patient prone: (a) Feel for tenderness, watching the patient's face for any reaction. (b) Performing the femoral stretch test. You can test for lumbar root sensitivity either by hyperextending the hip or by acutely flexing the knee with the patient lying prone. Note the point at which the patient feels pain and compare the two sides. (c) While the patient is lying prone, take the opportunity to feel the pulses. The popliteal pulse is easily felt if the tissues at the back of the knee are relaxed by slightly flexing the knee.

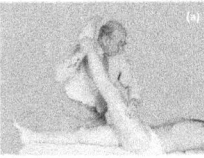 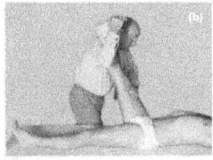 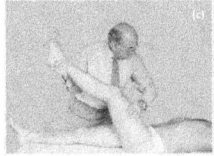 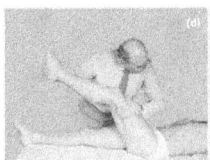

Sciatic stretch tests: (a) Straight-leg raising. The knee is kept absolutely straight while the leg is slowly lifted (or raised by the patient himself); note where the patient complains of tightness and pain in the buttock – this normally occurs around 80 or 90°. (b) At that point a more acute stretch can be applied by passively dorsiflexing the foot – this may cause an added stab of pain. (c) The 'bowstring sign' is a confirmatory test for sciatic tension. At the point where the patient experiences pain, relax the tension by bending the knee slightly; the pain should disappear. Then apply firm pressure behind the lateral hamstrings to tighten the common peroneal nerve (d); the pain recurs with renewed intensity.

4- ORTHOPEDIC EXAMINATION..

Neck *(Cervical spine)* examination:

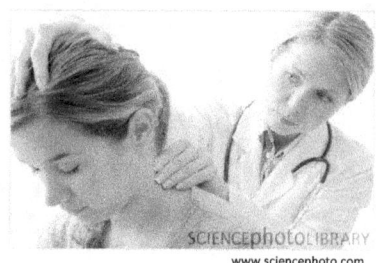

First: greet the patient,
introduce yourself,
take permission for examination,
hand washing,
make sure patient privacy,
good exposure *' trunk & both upper limbs '*

Look: *symmetry,* deformity, swelling or redness, ulcer, wasting, scar, sinus & skin lesions..

Feel: *' ask him if he has any pain '..* *(anterior → from behind, posterior → in prone position)*
temperature & spinous process for *tenderness & steps..*
finger breadth

Move: **active..** flexion (chin on chest → 75°), extension (look up at the ceiling → 60°),
rotation (look over your shoulder → 80°),
lateral flexion (put your ear on the shoulder → 45°)

Special tests: [in **THORACIC** spine examination → the *chest expansion* is the most important difference & the *ALL OTHER STEPS* are *THE SAME..*]

Don't forget: neurovascular examination & L.N. examination.. *(Allen's test is included..)*
Suggest to examine the distal joints..

At the end: cover the patient, thank him..

4- ORTHOPEDIC EXAMINATION..

*** References:** www.osceskills.com
Apley's System of Orthopaedics and Fractures

Some of helpful images for ' *Neck (Cervical spine) examination* ':

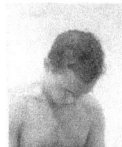 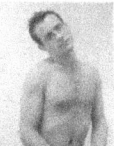 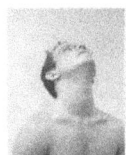 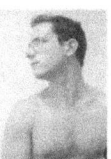

Flexion - movement   Flexion – movement 2   Extension - movement   Rotation - movement

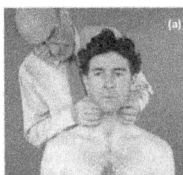 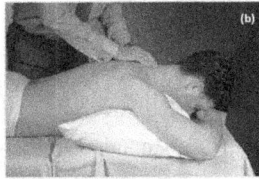 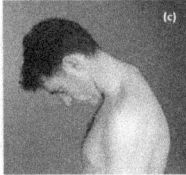 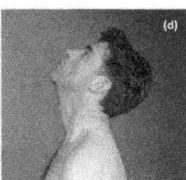

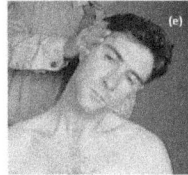 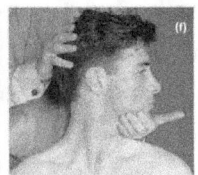

Examination: (a) The front of the neck is felt with the patient seated and the examiner standing behind him. (b) The back of the neck is most easily and reliably felt with the patient lying prone over a pillow; this way muscle spasm is reduced and the neck is relaxed. (c-f) Movement: flexion ('chin on chest'); extension ('look up at the ceiling'); lateral flexion ('tilt your ear towards your shoulder')' and rotation ('look over your shoulder').

4- ORTHOPEDIC RADIOLOGY..

How to report ' THE ORTHOPEDICS AND FRACTURES X-RAY ':

First: This is a *plain X-ray,* A-P view,
taking for *Suha Ramzi, 27 y. old,*
at the 25th of October 2012,
right or left ??..

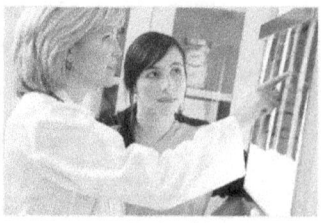
www.mydoctor.kaiserpermanente.org

Showing: *' check for any abnormality in.. '*

- The lower third of the Right thigh (femur), knee joint, upper part of tibia & fibula,
- Good quality of skeletally mature *(if epiphyseal plate is fused)..*
- *I don't accept this X-ray bec. It doesn't show the other view..etc (rule of 2),*
- There is a back slap from above the knee to ……
- Disrupted skin, shells in the subcutaneous, swelling & the muscle is normal,
- Any fracture → *describe it..*
- Any displacement → *describe it..*
- *Don't forget the proximal & distal joints..*

At the end: thank him..

FRACTURE:
- transverse
- oblique or spiral
- impacted
- green stick
- compression

DISPLACEMENT:
- shifted
- angulated
- overlapped
- impacted
- twisted

RULE OF 2:
- 2 *views* (A-P & Lat. for ex.)
- 2 *occasions* (after 10 days in scaphoid f. for ex.)
- 2 *limbs* (in children to compare with the other limb)
- 2 *joints* (proximal & distal)
- 2 *bones* (Radius & ulna for ex.)
- 2 *opinions* (2 doctors..)

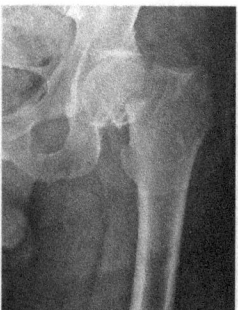
Femur neck fracture

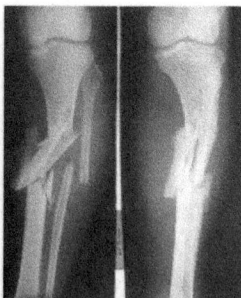
Tibia & fibula fracture

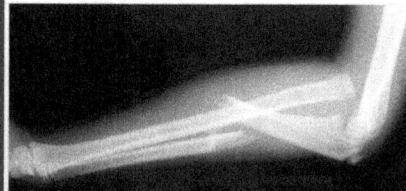
Monteggia fracture

CHAPTER 5

PEDIATRICS

Contents:

HISTORY TAKING
   CASE SHEETs   131
   Jaundice H_x 136
   Hematuria   137
   Fit H_x 138
   Enuresis H_x 139
   Joint swelling H_x 140
   Diabetes mellitus H_x 141
   Diarrhea H_x 142
   Wheezy chest H_x 143
   Cough H_x 144
   Fever H_x 145
   Cardiac disease H_x 146

EXAMINATION
   General Ex   147
   Respiratory distress Assessment   148
   Hydration status assessment   148
   Nutritional status assessment   149
   Patient with meningitis   150
   Patient with bleeding tendency   151
   Patient with diabetes   152
   Patient with jaundice   153
   Patient with Hematuria   154
   Patient with diarrhea   154
   Patient with edema (N.S.)   155
   Patient with hydrocephalus   156
   Patient with rickets   156
   Down syndrome   157
   Temperature measurement   157
   Height measurement in children   158

COMMUNICATION SKILLS
   Diabetes mellitus ' Insulin injection '   159
   Diabetes mellitus ' Diabetes diet '   160
   Diabetes M. ' Hypoglycemic attacks '   160
   Diabetes M. ' How to use a glucometer '   161
   Lumbar puncture   162
   Breast feeding   163
   Oral rehydration solution (O.R.S.)   165
   Enuresis   166
   Vaccination   167
   Vaccines   169

INVESTIGATIONS
   Normal values   171
   Cerebrospinal fluid (C.S.F.) analysis   172
   N. S. vs. Glumerilunephritis   173
   Trick - Hematology   174

FOLLOW UP CHARTS   175
DEVELOPMENT MADE VERY EASY   176
DRUGs ' ESSENTIAL NOTEs '   178
INTRAVENOUS FLUIDs   187
BLOOD PRODUCTs   189
OTHER IMPORTANT TOPICS
   Lumbar puncture   190
   Bone marrow aspiration & biopsy   190
   Exchange transfusion   191
   Phototherapy   192
   Ventolin nubulizar (Salbutamol)   192
   Different types of drips   193
   Intraousseous needle   193
   Liver biopsy   194
   Urine analysis (Urine dipstick)   194
   Other important topics   194

5- PEDIATRICS — HISTORY TAKING [CASE SHEET]..

HISTORY CASE SHEET :

DEMOGRAPHY DATA:

Name:
Date of birth & age :
Sex :
Address :
Date of admission:
Date of taking history :
Source of history : *(patient, mother or both of them ?)*

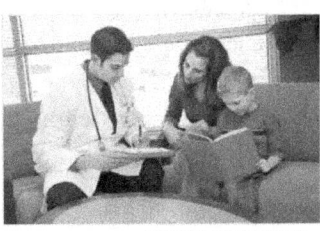

CHIEF COMPLAINT & DURATION:

H. OF PRESENT ILLNESS:

Ask about :

How and when the illness started (SYSTEM INVOLVED) ?

Any changes in the course of the illness ?

Any drugs are given ? any benefit ?

Mention the effect of illness on [THE SIX]:

Appetite ?

Weight ?

Bowel motion ?

Urine output ?

Sleep ?

Activity ?

Progress of illness in the hospital ?

SYSTEMS REVIEW :

Alimentary system & the abdomen:

Difficulty in swallowing : For liquids or with solid food ?
Food stuck ? Level ?

Regurgitation : How often ?
Aggravating factors ?
Heartburn ?
Vomiting : Any blood ?
Abdominal pain ? *(mention pain analysis)*
Abdominal distension ?

5- PEDIATRICS   HISTORY TAKING [CASE SHEET]..

Bowel motion : Diarrhea or constipation ?
Yellowish discoloration of sclera & skin ?
Diet : Type of food ? , Any food prevention ? , At what age did he start table food ?

Respiratory system :
Cough : In attacks ? , Whooping ?
Sputum ?
Nasal discharge ?
Shortness of breath :   At rest ? , At night ? , On exertion ?
        Any previous attack ?
        Associated symptoms : Cough ? , Increase body temperature ? ,
          Bluish discoloration of the lips, face or limbs ?
        Effect on feeding ?
        Any family H_x ?

Wheezing ?
Bluish discoloration of the lips, face or limbs ?
Chest pain : *(in appropriate age)*

Cardiovascular system :
Shortness of breath : At rest ? , At night ? , On lying flat ? , Effect on feeding ?
Awareness of heart beats *(palpitation)* ?
Chest pain ?
Pallor ?
Bluish discoloration of the lips ,face ,limbs ?
Ankle swelling ?

Genitourinary system :
Urine stream ?
Any blood with urine ?
Loin pain ? *(mention pain analysis)*
Burning micturition ?
Testicular swelling ?
Puffy face, ankle swelling or abdominal distension ?
Shortness of breath ?

Nervous system :
Fits : Duration of complaint ?
   Date of 1st fit ? & Duration ?
   No. of fits /day ?
   What happen before & after it ?
   Child's condition between attacks ?
   Associated symptoms : Loss of consciousness ? , Tongue bite ?, Frothy secretion ?,
         Rolling of the eyes ? , Loss of sphincter control ? ,
         Verbalization ?

5- PEDIATRICS   HISTORY TAKING [CASE SHEET]..

Headache ?
Change in behavior ?
Change in activity ?
Change in gait or posture ?
Blurred vision ?

Chocking & cough with feeding ?

Locomotor system :
Limping ?
Limb swelling or pain ?
Bruises ?
Any deformity ?

ANTENATAL Hx:

Maternal health before and during pregnancy ?
Attend antenatal care clinic regularly ?
H_x of D.M. , Hypertension , Anemia or Bleeding ?
H_x of infection *(TORCH)*, Fever , Rash , Cervical swellings ?
Any drug use ?
Smoking or Alcohol ?
H_x of leaking liquor ?
Toxoid vaccine ?

Natal Hx:

Normal vaginal bleeding or caesarian section ? Why ?
Difficulties & length of labor ?
Any analgesia was given ?
Any resuscitation ?
Cry immediately ? , Breath spontaneously ?
Pass meconium ?

Birth order ? , Birth weight ?
Gestational age ?

Postnatal Hx:

Admission to ICU or delivered to mother ?
H_x of jaundice , H_x of photo-therapy , H_x of blood exchange ?
Fit ?
Fever ?

5- PEDIATRICS — HISTORY TAKING [CASE SHEET]..

PAST-MEDICAL Hx:

Any communicable disease : As Chickenpox , Mumps , Measles , Whooping cough or Chronic disease like D.M.
Previous hospitalization : in E.R. ?

DRUG Hx:

Take any drugs ?
Allergy to drug ?
Allergy to food ?

PAST-SURGICAL Hx:

Any previous operation ?
Anesthesia ?
Blood exchange ?

FAMILY Hx:

FATHER & MOTHER → Age ? , Jobs ? , Health condition ? & Consanguinity ?
SIBLING → NO. ? , Age ? , Health condition ?
Hx of Asthma , Eczema , Cardiovascular illness … etc. ?
Any similar illness in the family ?
Hx of death in the family ?

SOCIO-ECONOMIC Hx:

Environment (rural or urban) ?
Water sanitation ?
Overcrowding in home (No. of people in the room) ?
Smokers in the home ?
Animal (pets) ?
Income of the family ?

VACCINATION Hx:

Date & Site of vaccination ?
Check the schedule (Vaccination program in Iraq) ?
Sever reaction after vaccination ?
Date of last vaccine ?

5- PEDIATRICS — HISTORY TAKING [CASE SHEET]..

FEEDING Hx:

    Type : (Breast , Bottle , mixed) or solid food ?
        If bottle feeding → Why shift to bottle feeding ?
                            Frequency ?
                            Amount & duration ?
                            Good bottle sterilization ?
                            Date of introducing solid food ?

        If breast feeding → Frequency ?
                              Duration of feed ?
                              Any difficulties ?
                              Exclusive or not ?

DEVELOPMENTAL Hx:

    (Milestone) ?? → *See page no. 176*

5- PEDIATRICS — focus HISTORY TAKING..

Jaundice ' history taking ':

FIRST: greet the mother,
introduce yourself,

START WITH DEMOGRAPHY:

name, date of birth, sex, address,
date of admission & date of taking H_x, source of H_x..

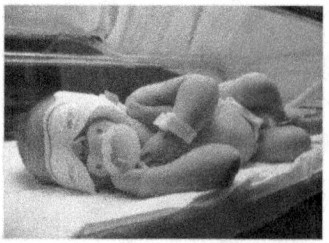

CHIEF COMPLAINT & DURATION:

H_x OF PRESENT ILLNESS:

onset, at which day start ?, color of jaundice (lemon or green),

urine & stool color, **itching**, fever, convulsion, pallor or bleeding,

[weight, appetite, bowel motion, urine output, activity & sleep] = [THE 6]

↓↓ level of consciousness & fit (C.N.S.), abnormal behavior & school performance..

then complete the gastrointestinal system H_x (frequent vomiting is very important)..

PAST MEDICAL H_x: bleeding, blindness or neuropathy (due to vit. K,E,D & A deficiency)..
PAST SURGICAL H_x:
DRUG H_x: ASNANK (aspirin, sulfa drugs, nitrofurantoin, anti-malarial, nalidixic acid, Vit.K) or depakin..

FAMILY H_x: mother & father blood group & Rh, similar condition, abortion or H_x of death due to similar condition in the family..
SOCIOECONOMIC H_x: sanitation, pets..

ANTENATAL CARE H_x: take blood or plasma, had any fever or rash..
NATAL H_x: preterm ?, 1st child, normal vaginal delivery (N.V.D.) or by C/S..
POST-NATAL H_x: take exchange transfusion or photoR_x ?, delay passage of meconium..

VACCINATION H_x: HBV vaccine ??
FEEDING H_x: bottle or breast, ingestion of fova beans..
DEVELOPMENTAL H_x: vision (head fixation & follow mother face), social smile ..etc

& don't forget the REVIEW of SYSTEMS:

At the end: thank the mother..

5- PEDIATRICS — focus HISTORY TAKING..

Hematuria ' history taking ':

FIRST: greet the mother & the patient,
introduce yourself,

START WITH DEMOGRAPHY:

name, date of birth, sex, address,
date of admission & date of taking H_x, source of H_x..

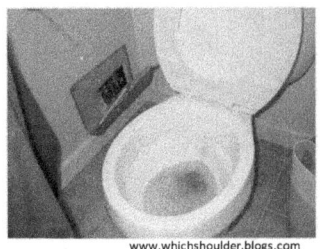

www.whichshoulder.blogs.com

CHIEF COMPLAINT, ONSET & DURATION:

H_x OF PRESENT ILLNESS:

skin infection before few weeks *or* upper respiratory tract infection before few days..,

frequency, urgency or painful micturition..

amount & color of urine,

body swelling, abdominal or flank pain, fever or rash,

bleeding, hemoptysis, stool color, trauma or heavy exercise..

loss of consciousness (encephalopathy) or headache,

[weight, appetite, bowel motion, urine output, activity & sleep] = [THE 6]

PAST MEDICAL H_x: photosensitivity ?
PAST SURGICAL H_x:
DRUG H_x:

FAMILY H_x: sickle cell disease..
SOCIOECONOMIC H_x:

*Trick: Don't forget the H_x must be in the patient words..
So, instead of Hematuria → we say red color urine
& so on.. [this is a general important note..]*

ANTENATAL CARE H_x:
NATAL H_x:
POST-NATAL H_x:

VACCINATION H_x:
FEEDING H_x:
DEVELOPMENTAL H_x:

& don't forget the REVIEW of SYSTEMS: ' if > 12 y. old → the *menstrual H_x* is very important '

At the end: thank the mother..

5- PEDIATRICS — focus HISTORY TAKING..

Fit ' history taking ':

FIRST: greet the mother,
introduce yourself,

START WITH DEMOGRAPHY:
name, date of birth, sex, address,
date of admission & date of taking H_x, source of H_x..

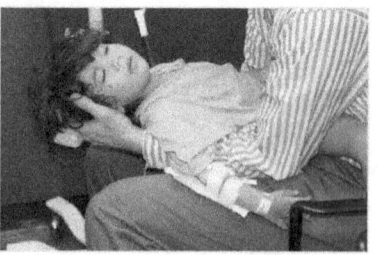

CHIEF COMPLAINT & DURATION:

H_x OF PRESENT ILLNESS:

onset, frequency, time of first fit ?, *What happen before the fit ?*

describe the attack → generalized, focal, tonic, or clonic, abnormal eye movements, drooling of saliva, verbalization, tongue bite, bluish discoloration, blurred vesion, incontinence or abnormal behavior..

trauma, diarrhea, fever or loss of consciousness, any aggravated factors..

what happen after attack ?, how to stop the attack?,

[weight, appetite, bowel motion, urine output, activity & sleep] = [THE 6]

then complete the C.N.S. system H_x

PAST MEDICAL H_x:
PAST SURGICAL H_x:
DRUG H_x:

FAMILY H_x: similar condition in the family ?
SOCIOECONOMIC H_x:

ANTENATAL CARE H_x: D.M. or T.O.R.C.H..
NATAL H_x: any complication, preterm, delay crying & meconium aspiration..
POST-NATAL H_x: jaundice..

VACCINATION H_x: pertusis, MMR..
FEEDING H_x:
DEVELOPMENTAL H_x: (IMPORTANT..)

& don't forget the REVIEW of SYSTEMS: it is very important especially the respiratory & cardiovascular systems

At the end: thank the mother..

5- PEDIATRICS — focus HISTORY TAKING..

Enuresis ' history taking ':

FIRST: greet the mother & the patient,
introduce yourself,

START WITH DEMOGRAPHY:
name, date of birth, sex, address,
date of admission & date of taking H_x, source of H_x..

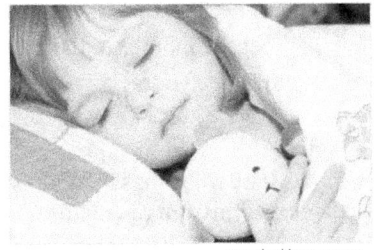
www.healthterrace.com

CHIEF COMPLAINT & DURATION:

H. OF PRESENT ILLNESS:

previously toilet trained or never attained control ? (1° or 2° ?)

frequency (how many time per day & per week), at daytime or at night ?,

sleep after that ?

ask about the urine & complete the urinary system (in day time)..

fluid intake, emotional stress (family problems..etc)

[THE 6]..

PAST MEDICAL H.: D.M., mental retarded, U.T.I or any renal abnormality..
PAST SURGICAL H.:
DRUG H.:

FAMILY H.: similar condition in the family ?
SOCIOECONOMIC H.:

ANTENATAL CARE H.:
NATAL H.:
POST-NATAL H.:

VACCINATION H.:
FEEDING H.:
DEVELOPMENTAL H.:

& don't forget the REVIEW of SYSTEMS:

At the end: thank the mother..

5- PEDIATRICS — focus HISTORY TAKING..

Bleeding tendency ' history taking ':

FIRST: greet the mother & the patient,
introduce yourself,

START WITH DEMOGRAPHY:
name, date of birth, sex, address,
date of admission & date of taking H_x, source of H_x..

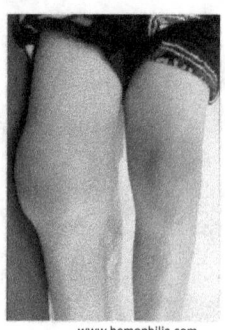
www.hemophilia.com

CHIEF COMPLAINT & DURATION:

H_x OF PRESENT ILLNESS:

site → skin, mucous mm, deep joints & mm., GIT, urine color

severity, spontaneous or after trauma ?, correlation with the degree of injury

pallor, fever, bone pain, joint swelling

other autoimmune disease?

Type of bleeding → patechae, echymmosis, hematoma & their sites, no., shape & color..

Jaundice? or headache, blurred vision (intracranial hemorrhage)

[THE 6]..

PAST MEDICAL H_x: previous attack, any I_x (BT, PT, PTT, CBC, platelets function test, TT, clotting factors, mixing study)..

PAST SURGICAL H_x: tonsillectomy, circumcision, dental procedure? & take plasma, cryo or platelets ?

DRUG H_x: aspirin or wrfarin

FAMILY H_x: similar condition in the family

SOCIOECONOMIC H_x:

Trick: In joint swelling Hx. ask the following questions:
onset, which joints ?, no. of joints ?, is this the 1st attack ?,
fever, rash or weight loss & night sweating,
swelling or redness, early morning stiffness.
trauma. mouth ulcer & red eye..
pain & bleeding tendency Hx.
[the 6].

ANTENATAL CARE H_x:
NATAL H_x:
POST-NATAL H_x:

VACCINATION H_x: any bleeding or swelling at the site of vaccination..
FEEDING H_x:
DEVELOPMENTAL H_x:

& don't forget the REVIEW of SYSTEMS:

At the end: thank you..

5- PEDIATRICS — focus HISTORY TAKING..

Diabetes mellitus ' history taking ':

FIRST: greet the mother & the patient,
introduce yourself,

START WITH DEMOGRAPHY:
name, date of birth, sex, address,
date of admission & date of taking Hx, source of Hx..

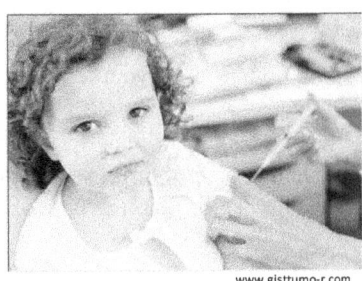
www.gisttumo-r.com

CHIEF COMPLAINT & DURATION:

Hx OF PRESENT ILLNESS:

onset, polyuria, nocturia, polydipsia, hyperphagia & weight loss,

for D.K.A → ***disturbed level of consciousness***, ***abdominal discomfort***, nausea & ***vomiting***, dehydration, weakness or ***deep heavy rapid respiration***..

↓↓ mentality ??

trauma.. stress ? or hypoglycemic attack or enuresis..

in ♀ patient → any abnormal discharge or itching..

[THE 6]..

PAST MEDICAL Hx: celiac disease, vitiligo, thyroid or S.L.E.
PAST SURGICAL Hx:
DRUG Hx: (IMPORTANT..)

FAMILY Hx: celiac disease..
SOCIOECONOMIC Hx: psychological stress..

ANTENATAL CARE Hx: rubella or maternal D.M.
NATAL Hx:
POST-NATAL Hx:

VACCINATION Hx:
FEEDING Hx:
DEVELOPMENTAL Hx:

Trick: Don't forget the Hx must be in the patient words..
So, instead of hyperphagia → we say increased consumption of food & so on.. [this is a general important note..]

& don't forget the REVIEW of SYSTEMS:

At the end: thank the mother..

5- PEDIATRICS   focus HISTORY TAKING..

Diarrhea ' history taking ':

FIRST: greet the mother & the patient,
introduce yourself,

START WITH DEMOGRAPHY:
name, date of birth, sex, address,
date of admission & date of taking H_x, source of H_x..

CHIEF COMPLAINT & DURATION:

H_x OF PRESENT ILLNESS:

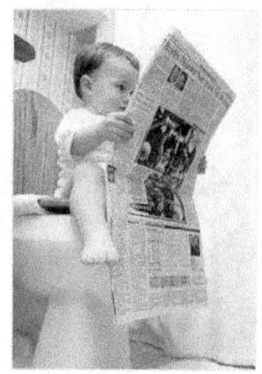

onset, amount, frequency, consistency & odor,

color, mucus or blood..

fever, abdominal pain or distension, vomiting or tensmus

related to feeding

then complete the gastrointestinal system H_x..

[THE 6]..

PAST MEDICAL H_x:
PAST SURGICAL H_x.
DRUG H_x: (IMPORTANT..)

FAMILY H_x: similar condition in the family ?
SOCIOECONOMIC H_x: water supply & sanitation..

ANTENATAL CARE H_x:
NATAL H_x:
POST-NATAL H_x:

VACCINATION H_x:
FEEDING H_x: bottle or breast feeding ?
DEVELOPMENTAL H_x:

& don't forget the REVIEW of SYSTEMS:

At the end: thank the mother..

5- PEDIATRICS — focus HISTORY TAKING..

Wheezy chest ' history taking ':

Trick: ' PEASE, SEE THE NEXT PAGE.. '

FIRST: greet the mother & the patient,
introduce yourself,

START WITH DEMOGRAPHY:
name, date of birth, sex, address,
date of admission & date of taking H_x, source of H_x..

CHIEF COMPLAINT & DURATION:

H_x OF PRESENT ILLNESS:

onset, increased at specific time ?,

cough (*especially after crying or at night*) or blush discoloration of the face & lips,

fever or vomiting..

foreign body aspiration ??

then complete the respiratory system H_x..

[THE 6]..

PAST MEDICAL H_x: eczema, any previous hospitalization ?
PAST SURGICAL H_x:
DRUG H_x:

FAMILY H_x: asthma, cystic fibrosis, immunodeficiency or similar condition in the family ?
SOCIOECONOMIC H_x: smokers at home ?, pet ?.. overcrowding ?

ANTENATAL CARE H_x:
NATAL H_x: gestational age ?, any intubation ?
POST-NATAL H_x:

VACCINATION H_x: (IMPORTANT..)
FEEDING H_x: any feeding difficulty ?, any new food exposure ?
DEVELOPMENTAL H_x:

& don't forget the REVIEW of SYSTEMS:

At the end: thank the mother..

5- PEDIATRICS   focus HISTORY TAKING..

Cough ' history taking ':

Trick: ' PLEASE, SEE THE PREVIOUS PAGE. '

FIRST: greet the mother & the patient,
introduce yourself,

START WITH DEMOGRAPHY:
name, date of birth, sex, address,
date of admission & date of taking H_x, source of H_x..

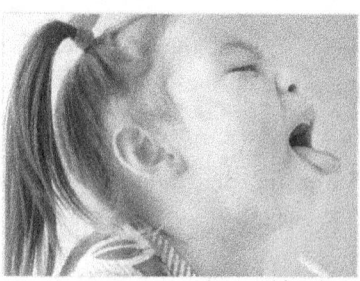

www.howtogetridofacough.org

CHIEF COMPLAINT & DURATION:

H_x OF PRESENT ILLNESS:

productive or not ?

frequency, continuous or intermittent ?, any diurnal variation ?

character ?..

any → chest pain, wheeze, bluish discoloration, change in the level of consciousness, fever or vomiting..

weight loss & sweating → [THE 6]..

PAST MEDICAL H_x:
PAST SURGICAL H_x:
DRUG H_x:

FAMILY H_x: similar condition in the family ?
SOCIOECONOMIC H_x: (IMPORTANT..)

ANTENATAL CARE H_x:
NATAL H_x:
POST-NATAL H_x:

VACCINATION H_x:
FEEDING H_x:
DEVELOPMENTAL H_x:

& don't forget the REVIEW of SYSTEMS:

At the end: thank the mother..

5- PEDIATRICS focus HISTORY TAKING..

Fever ' history taking ':

FIRST: greet the mother,
introduce yourself,

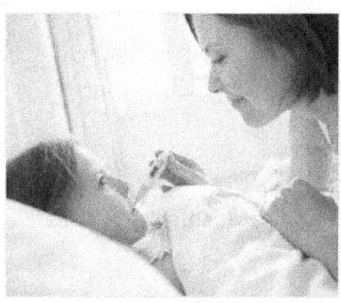

START WITH DEMOGRAPHY:
name, date of birth, sex, address,
date of admission & date of taking H$_x$, source of H$_x$..

CHIEF COMPLAINT & DURATION:

H$_x$ OF PRESENT ILLNESS:

continuous, intermitted or remitted, severity, sweating & shivering,

at specific time..   nausea or projectile..

relieving factors → drugs, antipyretic or cold sponge

associated symptoms → convulsion, blush discoloration of the face & lips, headache,

weight loss, rash, jaundice,

joint pain, swelling, warmth or stiffness..

[THE 6]..

PAST MEDICAL H$_x$:
PAST SURGICAL H$_x$:
DRUG H$_x$:

FAMILY H$_x$:
SOCIOECONOMIC H$_x$:

ANTENATAL CARE H$_x$ (IMPORTANT.. → fever, rash, ……. sexual transmitted disease)
NATAL H$_x$: (IMPORTANT.. → premature, prolonged rupture membrane & chorioamnionitis)
POST-NATAL H$_x$:

VACCINATION H$_x$:
FEEDING H$_x$:
DEVELOPMENTAL H$_x$:

& don't forget the REVIEW of SYSTEMS: (IMPORTANT..)
 (The important causes → U.T.I., meningitis, dysentery, joint & bone infection, sepsis)

At the end: thank the mother..

5- PEDIATRICS   focus HISTORY TAKING..

Cardiac diseases ' history taking ':

FIRST: greet the mother,
introduce yourself,

START WITH DEMOGRAPHY:
name, date of birth, sex, address,
date of admission & date of taking H_x, source of H_x..

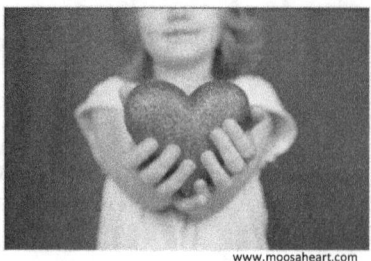
www.moosaheart.com

CHIEF COMPLAINT & DURATION:

H. OF PRESENT ILLNESS:

shortness of breath (during feeding, at night or when lying flat),

chest pain,

bluish discoloration of the face & lips,

fatigue or leg swelling,

failure to thrive → [THE 6]..

PAST MEDICAL H.:
PAST SURGICAL H.:
DRUG H.:

FAMILY H.: heart problems or similar condition in the family ?
SOCIOECONOMIC H.:

ANTENATAL CARE H.: gestational D.M., medication, S.L.E., substance abuse or maternal rubella..

NATAL H.: premature, bluish discoloration of the face & lips or respiratory distress..
POST-NATAL H.:

VACCINATION H.:
FEEDING H.: any difficulty ?, frequency..
DEVELOPMENTAL H.:

& don't forget the REVIEW of SYSTEMS:

At the end: thank the mother..

5- PEDIATRICS — EXAMINATION..

General examination:

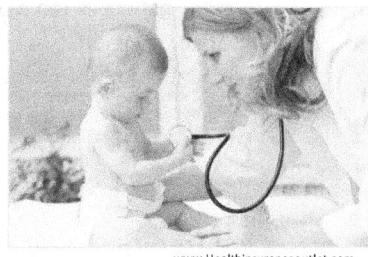

- **First:** greet the patient & the mother,
  introduce yourself,
  take permission for examination,
  hand washing,
  make sure patient privacy,
  good exposure *' when needed..'*

- **General look:** *' for example '*, a ♀ infant, lying flat in the bed,
  she look well, comfortable, conscious, alert, oriented *(for place, person and time),*
  not dyspneic, no wheeze & no stridor,
  no dysmprphic features & no specific complexion,
  with yellow i.v. cannula in her right hand, no i.v. fluid, no O_2 bottle ….etc

- **Head:** anterior fontanelle *(sitting & quite),*
  eye → jaundice, pallor, tear, conjunctival hemorrhage, pre-orbital edema & malar rash,
  ear → low set ears ?
  nose → nasal flaring,
  lips & mouth → cyanosis, jaundice, pallor, angular stomatitis, moist ?, thrush,
  gum (any bleeding ?), tongue, tonsils & palate..

- **Neck:** L.N. & thyroid gland..

- **Hand:** pallor, cyanosis, clubbing, edema, splinter hemorrhage, hot & sweating,
  palmer erythema, koilonychias, any deformity or Osler's nodes..

- **Arm & forearm:** radial pulse *(vital signs)* & skin lesions (rash, bruises, hematoma, petechiae,
  vitiligo & café au lait),

- **Axilla:** L.N.

- **Chest:** inspection → deformity, movement ..etc, **[signs of respiratory distress]..**

- **Abdomen:** distention..etc, skin turgor **[nutritional assessment]..**

- **Lower limb & Genitalia:** edema, skin lesion, joint swelling, deformity, inguinal L.N.,
  , genitalia & napkin area → *dermatitis, stool & ambiguous genitalia..*

- **Don't forget:** *[Nutritional assessment], [Dehydration assessment], [Growth parameters]..*

- **At the end:** cover the patient & thank the mother.. ↖ Trick: This is an important step in the all next topics..

5- PEDIATRICS — EXAMINATION..

Respiratory distress assessment:

First: greet the patient & the mother,
introduce yourself,
take permission for examination,
hand washing,
make sure patient privacy,
good exposure *' when needed..'*

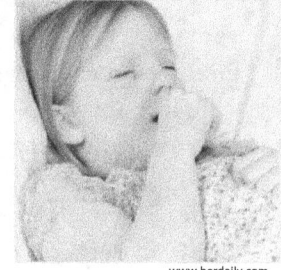

Then examine: consciousness,
wheeze, grunting, stridor,
alar nose flaring,
cyanosis,
retraction (suprasternal, intercostals & subcostal),
use of accessory muscles,
vital signs (respiratory rate..),
complete chest examination..

At the end: cover the patient & thank the mother..

Hydration status assessment:

First: greet the patient & the mother,
introduce yourself,
take permission for examination,
hand washing,
make sure patient privacy,
good exposure *' when needed..'*

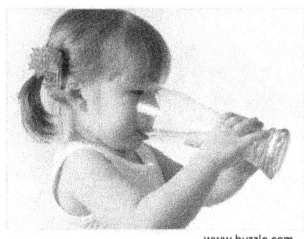

*Then examine: consciousness,
eager to drink,
skin turgor,*
fontanelle (depressed ?),
eye (sunken ?, tears ?),
mouth (dry ?),
capillary refilling (press on the sternum 5 sec.),
urine output,
vital signs & growth parameters..

At the end: cover the patient & thank the mother..

5- PEDIATRICS — EXAMINATION..

Nutritional status assessment:

First: greet the patient & the mother,
introduce yourself,
take permission for examination,
hand washing,
make sure patient privacy,
good exposure *' when needed..'*

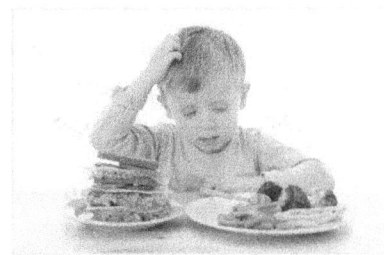
www.childrenssite.net

General look: apathy (kwashiorkor) or irritable (marasmus),

Signs of wasting: buttock,
inner thigh,
mid-upper arm circumference,
master muscles,

Edema:

Skin: wrinkling, pealing or darkening,

Mouth: angular stomatitis, tongue atrophy,

Growth parameters: OFC, weight, height,

Other: hair → flag sign in kwashiorkor, easily removed in marasmus..
orifices → acrodermatitis enteropathica..
signs of rickets or iron deficiency anemia..
liver enlargement..
abdominal distension..

At the end: cover the patient & thank the mother..

★★ For cardiovascular system, respiratory, nervous, G.I.T. systems examination, you can see chapter ' 1 '.. *(with some differences because the child may be not compliant in some steps)..*

5- PEDIATRICS — EXAMINATION..

Patient with meningitis:

First: greet the patient & the mother,
introduce yourself,
take permission for examination,
hand washing,
make sure patient privacy,
good exposure *'when needed..'*

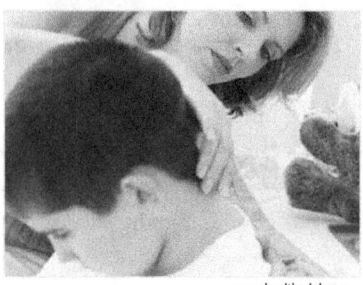
www.healthadel.com

General: consciousness, posture & skin,

Vital signs:

Meningeal signs:

Fontanelle & OFC + Pupil & fundoscopy:

Neuro-examination: cranial nerves,
upper & lower limbs,

Then: complete the growth parameters..

At the end: cover the patient & thank him..

5- PEDIATRICS — EXAMINATION..

Patient with bleeding tendency (or pallor):

First: greet the patient & the mother,
introduce yourself,
take permission for examination,
hand washing,
make sure patient privacy,
good exposure ' *when needed..* '

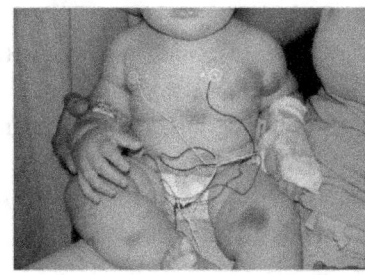
www.chla.org

General look:

Head: pallor & jaundice,
L.N.
subconjunctival hemorrhage, gum bleeding, tongue, lips, fontanelle & fundoscopy,

Neck: L.N.

Hand: pallor, nail-bed, cyanosis, clubbing,
palmer erythema, koilonychias,
cannula site,

Arm & forearm: radial pulse (*vital signs*),
skin lesions (rash ' *fade with pressure* ', bruises, hematoma or petechiae),

Axilla: L.N.

Chest: spider nevi & heart auscultation.

Abdomen: especially for hepatosplenomegaly,

Legs: edema & *joints swelling*,

Neurological examination: especially the reflexes (Babinski).

You can see: the urine & stool color, if there is any sample..

At the end: cover the patient & thank the mother..

5- PEDIATRICS — EXAMINATION..

Patient with diabetes:

First: greet the patient & the mother,
introduce yourself,
take permission for examination,
hand washing,
make sure patient privacy,
good exposure *'when needed..'*

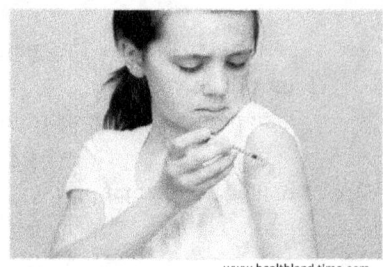

General look: consciousness, hydration status & any dysmorphic features,

Growth parameters: weight & height,

Vital signs: respiratory rate, radial pulse & blood pressure & temperature,

Abdomen: distension,

Site of injection: lypohypertrophy,
Site of infection: interdigital spaces or vaginal infection,

Prayer sign:

Skin (vitiligo), thyroid & eye (cataract):

Look for any other complication..

At the end: cover the patient & thank the mother..

5- PEDIATRICS — EXAMINATION..

Patient with jaundice:

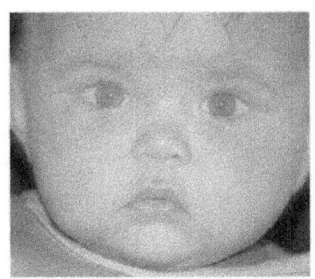

First: greet the patient & the mother,
introduce yourself,
take permission for examination,
hand washing,
make sure patient privacy,
good exposure '*when needed..*'

General look: consciousness & dysmorphic features,

Head: jaundice & pallor,
Scalp for hematoma, cataract,

Neck: L.N.

Hand: pallor, nail bed, clubbing, palmer erythema & cyanosis,

Arm & forearm: radial pulse (*vital signs*),
skin lesions (rash '*fade with pressure*', bruises, hematoma or petechiae),

Axilla: L.N.,

Chest: spider nevi,

Abdomen: compete examination.. (*especially for hepatosplenomegaly* & umbilical hernia),

Legs: edema,

Napkin area: for stool & urine color..

You can see: the urine & stool color, if there is any sample..

Don't forget: [*Nutritional assessment*], [*Dehydration assessment*], [*Growth parameters*],
[*primitive reflex (moro reflex)*]..

At the end: cover the patient & thank the mother..

5- PEDIATRICS — EXAMINATION..

Patient with hematuria:

First: greet the patient & the mother,
introduce yourself,
take permission for examination,
hand washing,
make sure patient privacy,
good exposure *' when needed..'*

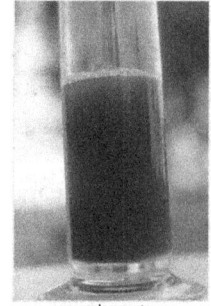

General look:

Head: tonsils, malar rash & periorbital edema,

Hand:
Arm & forearm: radial pulse & B.P. (*vital signs*),
skin lesions (rash ' *fade with pressure* ', bruises, hematoma or petechiae),

Abdomen: renal mass & renal angle tenderness,

Genitalia: infection or truma

At the end: cover the patient & thank the mother..

Patient with diarrhea:

First: greet the patient & the mother,
introduce yourself,
take permission for examination,
hand washing,
make sure patient privacy,
good exposure *' when needed..'*

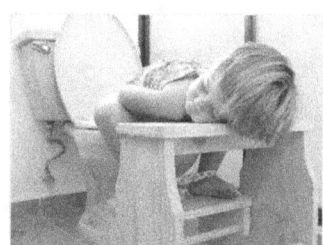

General look:
Dehydration status:
Nutritional status:
Growth parameters:

Vital signs:
Look for any signs of infection: (*otitis media, tonsillitis, U.T.I or viral..*)
Napkin area:

At the end: cover the patient & thank the mother..

5- PEDIATRICS — EXAMINATION..

Patient with edema (Nephrotic syndrome):

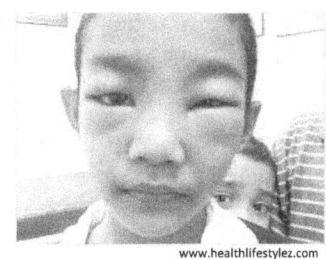
www.healthlifestylez.com

First: greet the patient & the mother,
introduce yourself,
take permission for examination,
hand washing,
make sure patient privacy,
good exposure *' when needed..'*

General look: periorbital puffiness,
leg edema,
abdominal distension,

Leg: edema,
pigmintation (*to differentiate between Kwashorkor & Nephrotic syndrome*),

Abdomen: ascitis (*shifting dullness & transmitted thrill*)

Chest: plural effusion,

Arm & forearm: swelling,

Genitalia: swelling,

Side effect of steroid:

Vital signs:

Don't forget: *[Nutritional assessment],*
[Growth parameters],

At the end: cover the patient & thank the mother..

Trick: Whenever you want to *touch the patient,* you have to ask him if he has any pain & you have to look to his face ' to observe his facial expression '..

Trick: Steroid S.E. ' CUSHING MAP ':

C → cataract, cushing's syndrome (iatrogenic)
U → peptic ulcer
S → stria
H → hirsutism, hyperglycemia, hypertension
I → infection, ↓↓ immunity, insomnia
N → necrosis of femoral head (avascular necrosis)
G → growth retardation
S → psychosis
M → myopathy (proximal type)
A → acne, acute adrenal failure (after sudden withdrawal)
P → porosis (osteo-), pancreatitis

5- PEDIATRICS — EXAMINATION..

Patient with hydrocephalus:

First: greet the patient & the mother,
introduce yourself,
take permission for examination,
hand washing,
make sure patient privacy,
good exposure *'when needed..'*

General look:

OFC: take 3 measures & consider the largest number.
Fontanelle & sun set eyes:
Sutures & dilated veins:
Transillumination:
Cracked pot sign: when you tap on the skull → abnormal sound..

for ↑↑ I.C.P.: examine the (vital signs, papilledema & cranial nerves),
Ventriculoperitoneal shunt: examine the course of the shunt..

At the end: cover the patient & thank the mother..

Patient with rickets:

First: greet the patient & the mother,
introduce yourself,
take permission for examination,
hand washing,
make sure patient privacy,
good exposure *'when needed..'*

General look:

Wide fontanelle:
Craniotabes: (The bone is soft and when pressure is applied they will collapse underneath it. When the pressure is relieved, the bones will usually snap back into place).
Bossing:
Teeth:
Rachitic rosary:
Harrison's sulcus: (*subcostal*)
Widening of radial & ulnar ends:
Bow legs & delayed walking:
Abdominal examination:

At the end: cover the patient & thank the mother..

5- PEDIATRICS — EXAMINATION..

Down syndrome (trisomy 21):

First: greet the patient & the mother,
introduce yourself,
take permission for examination,
hand washing,
make sure patient privacy,
good exposure *' when needed..'*

General look:

Head: flat occiput,
flat facial profile,
excess nuchal skin,
fontanelle,
slanted palpebral fissure, epicanthal fold, brushfield spot in eyes,
low set ears,
small jaw,

Hand: single crease (*simian crease*), short thick fingers & 5th finger dysplasia,

Legs: flat achillis tendon & crease between the 1st & 2nd toes (apes' groove)..

Nervous system examination: hypotonia, frog like posture & poor neonatal reflexes,

Chest: heart auscultation,

Abdominal examination:

At the end: cover the patient & thank the mother..

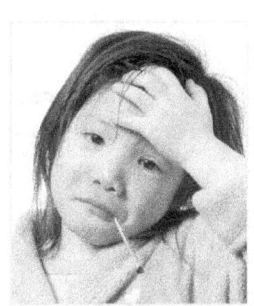

Temperature measurement:

The mercury thermometer degrees: 35 - 42 °C

Route: Oral,
Axillary corrected (+ 0.5° C) *' Safest '*,
Rectally corrected (- 0.5° C),
Aural..

Normal body temperature is: 36.5 - 37.5 °C

Trick: Don't touch this side, because..
- it is infectious side..
- may change the measurement..

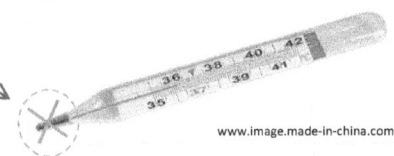

5- PEDIATRICS — EXAMINATION..

Height measurement in children:

First: greet the patient & the mother,

introduce yourself,

take permission for examination,

hand washing,

make sure patient privacy,

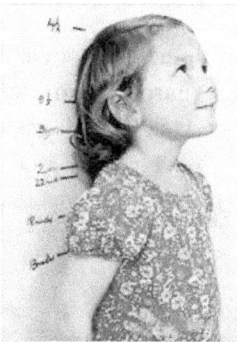

Then:
1. Remove the child's shoes, bulky clothing, and hair ornaments, and unbraid hair that interferes with the measurement.

2. Take the height measurement on flooring that is not carpeted and against a flat surface such as a wall with no molding.

3. Have the child stand with feet flat, together, and against the wall. Make sure legs are straight, arms are at sides, and shoulders are level.

4. Make sure the child is looking straight ahead and that the line of sight is parallel with the floor.

5. Take the measurement while the child stands with head, shoulders, buttocks, and heels touching the flat surface (wall). (See illustration.) Depending on the overall body shape of the child, all points may not touch the wall.

6. Use a flat headpiece to form a right angle with the wall and lower the headpiece until it firmly touches the crown of the head.

7. Make sure the measurer's eyes are at the same level as the headpiece.

8. Lightly mark where the bottom of the headpiece meets the wall. Then, use a metal tape to measure from the base on the floor to the marked measurement on the wall to get the height measurement.

9. Plot the result on the chart..

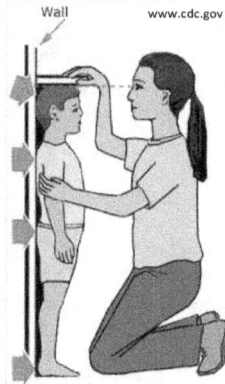

5- PEDIATRICS — COMMUNICATION SKILLS..

Trick: *'You have to use the country native language..'*

Diabetes mellitus 'Insulin injection':

INSULIN INJECTION: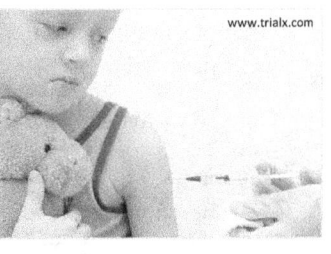

Greet the mother & introduce yourself,
Take permission..

There are *2 types* of syringes (even and odd)..
There are *3 types* of insulin (soluble, lente & mixed)..

The even syringe:
  Each line equivalent to **two** units of insulin,
    (between no.0 and number 10 there are only **five** lines)..

The odd syringe:
  Each line equivalent to **one** units of insulin,
    (between no.0 and number 10 there are **ten** lines)..

*You have to draw up the **soluble** insulin before the insoluble..*

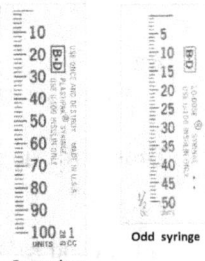
Even syringe   Odd syringe

Sites of injections → outer arm, abdomen, outer thigh & hip area.. [*subcutaneously*]..
  Injection is either by 45° or by a lifted skin fold method (lift the skin between thumb and two fingers with one hand, pulling the skin and fat away from the underlying muscle, and holding until the insulin has been injected)..

The site *should be changed* at each injection (rotated) to reduce the risk of skin thickness (lipohypertrophy) developing. A simple way to reduce this risk is to systematically rotate the site where the insulin is injected..

Change to another site..

INSULIN: There are **3 types** of insulin :
  Soluble (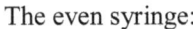, clear solution), lente (light blue or green vial, cloudy),
    mixed (brown, written on it *30 \ 70*)..
  You have to keep it in the refrigerator (but not in freeze), because it is a protein (damaged by heat)..

DOSE CALCULATION: '*according to age & weight*'
  Weight X **0.7** = no. of insulin units (2/3 at the morning, 1/3 at evening),
                                (1/3 soluble, 2/3 lente)..
  For example, if the child's weight is 21.5 kg. → he need 21.5 X **0.7** = 15 units of insulin..
            (10 unit at the morning, 5 at evening), (1/3 soluble, 2/3 lente)..

You have to plot a chart (date & time, blood sugar reading & insulin dose..)

AT THE END: thank the mother..

Diabetes mellitus 'Diabetes diet':

Greet the mother & introduce yourself,
Take permission..

Daily, 3 meals & 3 snacks..

Sugars (55%):
   Table sugar is forbidden..
   Potato, rice & breads → You have to choose one in each meal & reduce its amount..
   Fruits → one piece each day..

Fat (30%):
   Use vegetable oils only..

Proteins (15%):
   Use white meat only.. (*red meat is forbidden..*)

Don't provide all kinds of food in the refrigerator..

After each dose of insulin, the child **should eat**..

If the child **refuses to dine** (*for example*), he **should not** take the evening dose of insulin..

If the child insists to eat something (chocolate for example) → he can, **but either after** taking a dose of insulin **or** going to run or play football (*it is just an example*)..

Always, keep something sweet in the child's pocket..

Thank the mother..

Diabetes mellitus 'hypoglycemic attacks':

Greet the mother & introduce yourself,
Take permission..

You have to know hypoglycemic attack symptoms & how to deal with it..
   mild: *pallor, sweating, tearfulness, irritability & aggression..*
   moderate: *drowsy, confusion & personality changes..*
   sever symptoms: *inability to seek help & seizures or coma..*

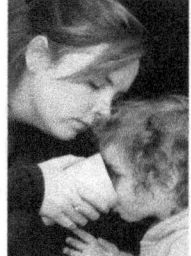

So, give him something sweet (*like an orange juice..*), then after 5 min, check the blood sugar [*if it is of no benefit or he can't drink* → inject him with glucagon..]

You have to plot a chart (date & time, blood sugar reading & insulin dose)..

Causes of hypoglycemia: Changed the person, the syringe or insulin type..
   Stress or sever exercise (*especially after the insulin dose*)..
   There is a gap between the insulin dose and the meal..
   Infection (hepatitis)..
   Nephropathy..

Thank the mother..

Trick: *'You have to use the country native language..'*

Diabetes mellitus ' How to Use a Glucometer ':

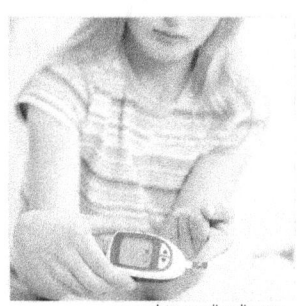
www.abcnewsradioonline.com

Greet the mother & the patient,
Introduce yourself,
Take permission..

Obtain a glucometer and test strips..

Wash the child hands thoroughly, including the area from which you are going to draw blood..

Place alcohol on a cotton ball..

Place a test strip into the slot provided on the glucometer..

Swab the area you are going to use to draw your sample from with the cotton ball..
  (Alcohol evaporates rapidly so there's no need to dry the area. That will just re-contaminate it)..

Wait for the readout on the diabetic glucometer to tell you to put the drop of blood on the strip..

Use the lancet provided with the diabetic glucose meter and prick the area for the sample..

Place a drop of blood on the test strip <u>without the finger touching the strip</u> & if touched the reading may be wrong *(and this is one of the techniqual errors that may occur)..*

Wait for results..

Read and record your results..
  You have to plot a chart *(date & time, blood sugar reading & insulin dose)..*

Thank the mother..

Trick: You can ask the mother if she has any questions, that will help you to remember if you forget any important information in the *communication skills OSCE* station or in your daily practical life..

Lumbar puncture:

Trick: 'You have to use the country native language.'

Greet the mother & the patient,
Introduce yourself,
Take permission..

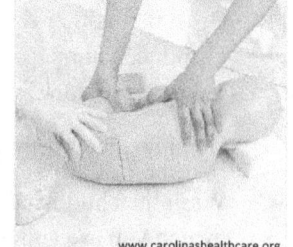

We suspect that your child has meningitis, which is a curable disease & its treatment is available..

But, to diagnose the disease we need a cerebral spinal fluid by a lumbar puncture.. it is simple, not danger prick like any prick of injection in the other body parts..

If she refuse..

The disease is dangerous and has a lot of complications like seizure, increase the intracranial pressure, paralysis & with time may loss his vision, hearing or even become mental retarded *(choose the simple complications & easy to understand by the mother)*..

If she refuses.. ' my relative was agree to do a lumbar puncture to his son which is know paralyzed !!, the mother said '..

O.K., believe me this is completely wrong, these are only rumors.. it is from other reason & not from the lumbar puncture itself..

If she insist to refuse the lumbar puncture..

O.K., we will give him an empirical treatment for 2 weeks, but we don't know whether it is the appropriate one or not (we will choose the most appropriate one).. and we follow his condition.. **BUT, believe me → the lumbar puncture is a right choice for his condition at this time (it is simple but worthy test)..**

Thank the mother..

5- PEDIATRICS — COMMUNICATION SKILLS..

Trick: 'You have to use the country native language..'

How to Sterilize & Prepare Baby Bottles:

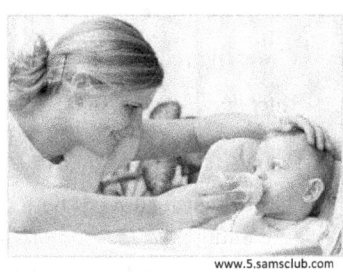

Greet the mother,
Introduce yourself,
Take permission..

Wash the bottle & nipple using water, table salt & with 2 brushes large one for bottle & small one for nipple..

Place a pot, filled with water, on the stove and turn the heat on to high till boiling..

Place the bottle in the water for **10 min.** (15 min. if glass bottle), then add the nipple to the water for **5 min.** → So, the full time is *15 min.* (20 min. if glass bottle)..

Turn off the stove, and wait till the water become cold.. (don't use cold water)..

Close the bottle and put it in the refrigerator..

When you want to prepare a milk baby bottle:
First, put the water in the bottle *then* add the milk..
Never dilute the milk..!!

Once no. calculation:
The ideal method (*according to weight*)..
Each 1 kg. need 100 k. calorie → So, **weight** X 100 = *no. of k. cal.* / day
There are 20 k.cal. in each ounce → So, **no. of k.cal.** / 20 = no. of ounce / day

For example.. the child weight is **4 kg**..
So, **4** X 100 = 400 k. cal. / day → 400 / 20 = **20 ounce / day**

The practical method (*according to weight*)..
Weight X 5 = No. of ounce
So, the previous example → 4 X 5 = **20 ounce / day**

[Ideally, the no. of bottles = no. feedings / day]..
And definitely, it is depend on the economic status of the family..

You may need to mention the advantages & disadvantages of the breast and bottle feedings to the baby and the mother..
(*please, see the next page..*)

Trick: Each one OUNCE = 30 ml.

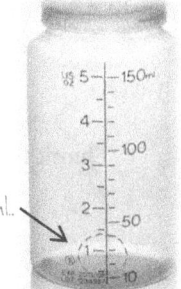

Therapeutic formula:
Soya based, CHO free milk & hydrolyzed protein formula
For specific medical purposes (like 1° & 2° lactase deficiency, galactosemia, fructosemia & cow milk protein intolerance)..

Thank the mother..

5- PEDIATRICS — COMMUNICATION SKILLS..

Trick: *'You have to use the country native language..'*

Breast feeding:

Greet the mother,

Introduce yourself,

Take permission..

The breast feeding is better than bottle feeding because the advantages *to the baby as well as to the mother..*
And don't forget, it is *easier, safer, cheaper & readily available..*
No milk allergy, has antimicrobial property, keep its gut sterile, and is consider the first natural vaccine you can give to the baby..
Also has proteins, fat, carbohydrates, water, vitamins & minerals..
Emotionally satisfactory for the mother & it gives feeling of security to the baby..

Rules of breast feeding:

Demand feeding & baby freedom..
↑↑ no. of feeding at night..
He should finish one breast then go to the other..
Rooming in or bedding in the same room..

*There are **no** real disadvantages of breast milk*, only we need to acknowledge them and deal with them immediately *(e.g.: inadequate lactation, demand maternal proximity, social life acceptance & treating cracked nipples by teaching the mother the technique of feeding)..*

Contraindication of breast feeding: '*most of them temporary*'

In mother: Sever systemic disease (acute heart failure, hepatitis B, neoplasia..etc)
　　　　　　Acute infection (active T.B., malaria, local bilateral breast abscesses..etc)
　　　　　　Insanity & uncontrolled epilepsy..
　　　　　　Sever inverted nipple not responding to local treatment..

In the baby: Iinborn error of metabolism *(absolute C.I.)..*
　　　　　　Sever physical abnormalities as bilateral cleft palate & cleft lip..
　　　　　　Weak & premature infant..　Sever dyspnoea as RDS & H.F.
　　　　　　Cerebral anoxia..

Thank the mother..

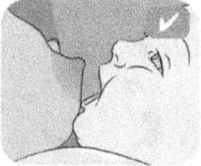 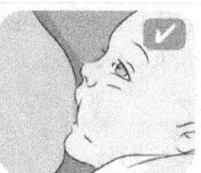 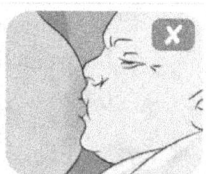

To start the feed, hold baby so her chest is touching your chest, her nose should be in line with your nipple. Gently brush your nipple from her nose to her upper lip – this will encourage her to open her mouth wide.

When her mouth is wide open, **bring baby to your breast** keeping your hands across her back and shoulders. When she attaches, most of the areola will be in her mouth and her chin will be tucked into the breast. When she's feeding well, she'll suck deeply and regularly, and you'll hear her swallowing.

When baby is not correctly attached and just sucks the nipple, feeding is painful, nipples can become damaged and the breast won't be properly drained. If baby hasn't attached correctly, stop, take her off the breast as shown below and try again.

www.abc.net.au

5- PEDIATRICS — COMMUNICATION SKILLS..

Trick: 'You have to use the country native language..'

Oral rehydration solution (O.R.S.):

Greet the mother,

Introduce yourself,

Take permission..

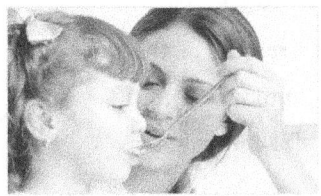

Your son has diarrhea.. but without dehydration yet..

So, *no* need for admission.. but you have to give him this solution *(Dextrolyte solution)*..

The child must continue his feeding (if he is breast fed to continue on feeding him with small frequent sips, if he is bottle fed to give fewer ounces but frequent times & if he is on diet to give him soft easily digestible diet in small amount and frequent times)..

Dissolve one pack in 1 liter of boiled water & wait till the water become cold then add the *Dextrolyte* solution..

It is given by spoon gradually to avoid acute gastric distension which causes vomiting & it is used for 24 h only..

For *below 24 months* → we give **50-100cc** of O.R.S. for each bowel motion passed and if the age *2-10 years* → we give **100-200 cc**..

If he vomits, we *wait for 10 minutes* and **then continue** giving the O.R.S by spoon but more slowly..

You have to bring the child to the 1° health care center if he is still having diarrhea after 2 days

Thank the mother..

Uses of O.R.S (DEXTROLYTE):
- It is given in acute diarrhea with **no dehydration** state to prevent dehydration..
- Also given for rehydration in **some dehydration** (mild to moderate) state..
- It is given for the **ongoing loss**..

Composition of O.R.S:
- NaCl → 3.5 g/l, NaHCO$_3$ → 2.5 g/l, KCl → 1.5 g/l, Glucose 20 g/l..

Concentration of O.R.S:
- Na$^+$ → 90 mmol/l, HCO$_3^-$ → 30 mmol/l, K$^+$ → 20 mmol/l, Cl$^-$ → 80 mmol/l & Glucose → 111 mmol/l..

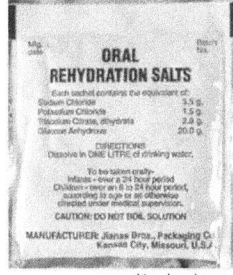

5- PEDIATRICS — COMMUNICATION SKILLS..

Trick: 'You have to use the country native language..'

Enuresis:

Greet the mother,

Introduce yourself,

Take permission..

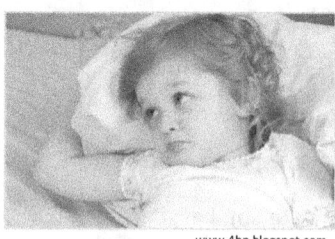

Doing nothing or punishing the child are both common responses to bedwetting. Neither helps.

You should reassure your child that bedwetting is common and can be helped.

Start by making sure that your child goes to the bathroom at normal times during the day and evening and does not hold urine for long periods of time.

Be sure that the child goes to the bathroom before going to sleep. You can reduce the amount of fluid the child drinks a few hours before bedtime, but this alone is not a treatment for bedwetting. You should not restrict fluids excessively.

Reward your child for dry nights. Some families use a chart or diary that the child can mark each morning.

Bedwetting alarms are another method that can be used along with reward systems. The alarms are small and readily available without a prescription at many stores.
The alarm wakes the child or parent when the child starts to urinate, so the child can get up and use the bathroom.

A prescription medication called DDAVP (desmopressin) is available to treat bedwetting.

Tricyclic antidepressants (most often imipramine) can also help with bedwetting.

Thank the mother..

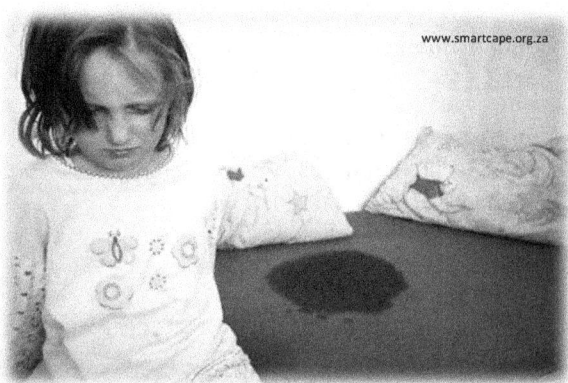

Don't forget - You should *reassure* the parents & the child that bedwetting is common and can be helped..

5- PEDIATRICS — COMMUNICATION SKILLS..

Trick: 'You have to use the country native language.'

Vaccination:

Greet the mother & introduce yourself,
Take permission..

Ask about → *Age* &
         The previous vaccination..

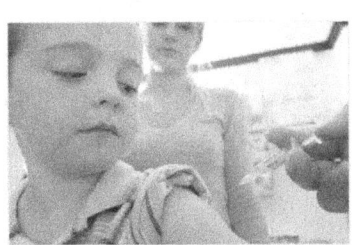

Vaccination schedule in Iraq:

    At birth → **BCG, OPV-0, HBV-1**
2 mo. completed → **DTP-1, OPV-1, HBV-2**   + *Rota virus & H. influenza vaccine*
4 mo. completed → **DTP-2, OPV-2,**   + *Rota virus & H. influenza vaccine*
6 mo. completed → **DTP-3, OPV-3, HBV-3**   + *Rota virus & H. influenza vaccine*
9 mo. completed → *Measles..*
15 mo. completed → *MMR..*
18 mo. completed → **DTP , OPV (booster no.1)** + *Vitamin A 200 I.U.*
  4-6 years → **DTP , OPV (booster no.2)** + *MMR 2*

What if a child misses a shot ?

    In the First visit → DTP-1, OPV-1, HBV-1   + *Rota virus & H. influenza vaccine*
          (± BCG)..

        1 mo. later → MMR..
    1-2 mo. later → DTP-2, OPV-2, HBV-2   + *Rota virus & H. influenza vaccine*
    1-2 mo. later → DTP-3, OPV-3, HBV-3   + *Rota virus & H. influenza vaccine*
15-18 mo. later → DTP , OPV **(booster)..**

NOTE: BCG vaccine is given to the baby in the first year to protect him from
      miliary T.B. & T.B. encephalitis → So, *after the 1st year is of NO benefit..*

Vaccination checklist: *(Be sure to ask these questions before giving the vaccines)..*

- Is your child **sick today** ? *(more than a common cold, earache ..etc)..*
- Does your child have any **sever** (life-threatening) **allergies** ?
- Has your child ever had **severe reaction after a vaccination** ?
- Does your child have a **weakened immune system** (bec. of disease or medication) ?
- Has your child **gotten a transfusion** or any other blood product, recently ?
  (if yes → wait 3 months..)..
- Has your child ever had **convulsion** or **any kind of nervous system problem** ?
- Does your child not seem to be **developing normally** ?

General contraindication for vaccination:

- Serious allergic reaction (*e.g.: anaphylaxis after a previous vaccine dose*)..
- Serious allergic reaction (*e.g.: anaphylaxis*) to a vaccine component..
- Moderate to severe illness with or without fever..

FALSE contraindication for vaccination:

- Mild acute illness with low grade fever or mild diarrhea..
- Mild to moderate local reaction (*soreness, redness or swelling*) after a dose of an injectable antigen..
- Current antimicrobial therapy..
- Prematurity..
- Malnutrition..
- Breast feeding..
- Pregnancy of mother or household contact..
- History of penicillin or other non specific allergy..
- Family H$_x$ of convulsion in child considered for pertussis or measles vaccination..
- Current antimicrobial therapy..

Vaccination in immunecompromised child: (*e.g.: with cancer or taking steroid*)..

- B̶C̶G̶, M̶M̶R̶, O̶P̶V̶ & R̶o̶t̶a̶ v. (*live attenuated*) → are CONTRAINDICATED..
- Give **HBV**..

Vaccination in pregnancy:

- B̶C̶G̶, M̶M̶R̶, O̶P̶V̶ & R̶o̶t̶a̶ v. (*live attenuated*) → are CONTRAINDICATED..
- Give **tetanus toxoid**..
  (At the 4th & the 5th months of pregnancy, then after 6 mo., 1 year, & 2 years)..

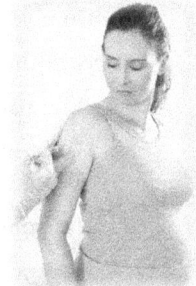

Why we give the vaccine according to the schedule ?

Answer: because at this time the immune system is mature enough to make the antibodies.. otherwise it is with no benefit..

AT THE END: thank the mother..

5- PEDIATRICS — COMMUNICATION SKILLS..

Trick: 'You have to use the country native language..'

Vaccines: *(To be oriented..!!)*

BCG:

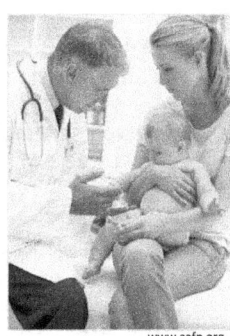

Is given as a single injection..
(intradermal + left side + at deltoid m. insertion).

A local abscess may form (BCG-oma) that may ulcerate & often requires treatment with antibiotic (erythromycin)..

Adverse effects → Keloids, large ugly scar (*main adverse effect*), Suppurative lymphadenitis (less common)..

If the mother refuse to give it to his child → *Explain to her that his child may become at risk of Miliary T.B. or T.B. encephalitis which are dangerous complication & lead to death..*

OPV:

Is given as oral drpos..

Adverse effects → on very rare occasions has been associated with paralysis (1 case per 750,000 vaccine recipient).. '*Don't mention this to the mother*'

If the mother refuse to give it to his child → *Explain to her that his child may become at risk of paralysis (may become unable to walk) & may affect on his respiration (may lead to death)..*

Hepatitis B vaccine:

Is given intramuscular as a three-dose series..
If the mother refuse to give it to his child → *Explain to her that his child may become at risk of hepatitis virus (which affect the liver functions)..*

DTP:

Is given intramuscular (0.5 ml)..
Adverse effects → minor: redness, swelling & painless nodule at the site of injection..
moderate: ongoing crying, high fever (up to 40) & unusual screaming..
severe: serious allergic reaction, seizures & encephalitis (very rare)..

If the mother refuse to give it to his child → *Explain to her that his child may become at risk of* : Pertussis: cough & respiratory problems → pneumonia (*most dangerous complication*)..
Diphtheria: may lead to respiratory & heart failure..
Tetanus: fever then spasms → may affect the respiratory system..

5- PEDIATRICS — COMMUNICATION SKILLS..

Trick: 'You have to use the country native language..'

MMR:

Greet the mother & introduce yourself,
Take permission..

Is given subcutaneously in two doses..

Adverse effects → fever & rash in 10% of children, 10 days after vaccine administration..
Transient arthritis & thrombocytopenia..

What are the benefits from this vaccine ?
  To protect the baby from measles, mumps & rubella..
  Rubella is given to ♀, not to protect her from rubella only but to prevent congenital rubella in pregnancy (to the baby if she get pregnant)..

If the mother refuse to give it to his child → *Explain to her that his child may become at risk of:*

  Rubella: Cause the same adverse effects of the vaccine but the commonest are arthralgia & arthritis..
  Measles: Cause fever, rash, influenza like symptoms, cough ..etc
    The commonest complication is otitis media but the dangerous one is 1° or 2° pneumonia..
  Mumps: Cause fever, influenza like symptoms, parotitis..etc
    The dangerous complication is meningitis.
    Orchitis is common in ♂ patients..

Thank the mother..

---

in / ARABIC /:

BCG = / LiL TADARON /,
OPV = / Li SHALAL al ATFAAL /,
H.B. vaccine = / Li ELTEHAB AL KABAD AL VAiROSee /

DTP → D (Diphtheria) = / AL KhANAK /,
     T (Tetanus) = / AL KOZAZZ /,
     P (Pertussis) = / AL So'AAL AL DEEKi /

MMR → M (Measles) = / AL HASBah /,
     M (Mumps) = / AL NOKAF /,
     R (Rubella) = / AL HASBah AL ALMANiAh /

Rota virus = / AL virus AL DAWAAR /,
H. influenza vaccine = / LiL MUSTADMIA AL NAZLiAA /,

INVESTIGATIONS..

Normal values:

WBC = 4 – 11 X 10^9/L,

Hb = 11 – 16 X g/dL,

Platelets = 150 – 400 X 10^9/L,

PCV = 37% – 47% in ♀ [Hb = (PCV-1) / 33]

Reticulocytes → < 2%

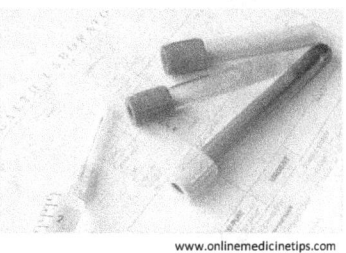

PT = 12 – 14 sec.

PTT = 30 – 45 sec.

TT = 10 – 13 sec. *' TT = Thrombin Time '*

BT = 4 – 8 min.

Reticulocytes = <2%

MCV:
80 - 95

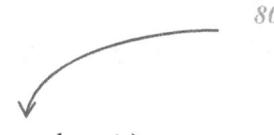

Less: *(microcytic hypochromic)*
 Iron deficiency anemia
 Thalassemia (major → Hb F >50%)
 Lead poisoning

More: *(macrocytic..)*
 Megaloblastic anemia
 B12 & folate deficiency

Normal: *(normocytic normochromic)*
 Hemolytic anemia
 Blood loss
 Renal disease
 ..etc

Cerebrospinal fluid (CSF) analysis:

Normal values:

Cells → <5 cell/mm² (75% lymphocytes),

Proteins = 20 – 45 mg/dL,

Glucose → > 50% mg/dL (75% of serum glucose)

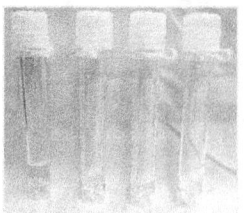

Meningitis:

	Pressure	Cells	Proteins	Glucose
Acute bacterial m.	N. or ↑↑	↑↑ polymorph.	↑↑	↓↓↓
Viral m.	N.	↑ Lymphocytes	N. / ↑↑	N.
T.B.	N. or ↑↑	↑ Lymphocytes	↑↑	↓↓
Partial Rₓ bacterial m.	N.	↑ Mononuclear	↑↑	N.

N. = normal, m. = meningitis

Guillain barré syndrome:

Albuminocytological dissociation (if the protein is only ↑↑ + oligoclonal band)..

Nephrotic syndrome Vs. Glumerilunephritis:

Nephrotic syndrome..   **Glumerilunephritis..**

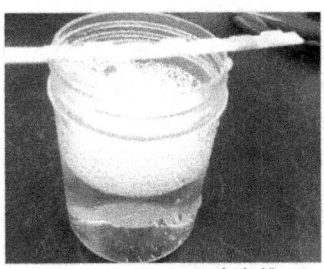 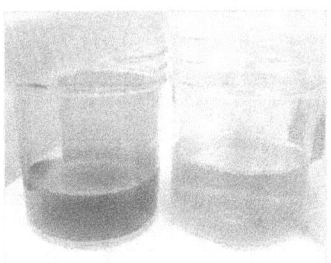

Normal color, frothy..   Red, macroscopic hematuria..

Proteins: +++ / ++++ (heavy proteinuria)   +

Casts: X   present

RBCs: X   > 5 (hematuria)

NOTE:

Normal serum albumin = 60 – 80 g/L..

5- PEDIATRICS — INVESTIGATIONS..

Trick:

This is the easiest way to memorize the HEMATOLOGY investigations, in general, not only in pediatrics.. !!

	ITP	TTP	E.T.
Platelets	↓ (< 80 × 10^9)	↓ (< 20 × 10^9)	↑ (600-2500 × 10^9)
B.T.	↑	↑	N.
PT	N.	N.	N.
PTT	N.	N.	N.
Bone marrow	N. or ↑↑ megakaryocyte	N. or ↑↑ cellularity	megakaryocytosis
Other I_x	Antiplatelet Ab +ve..	WBC ↑↑ gingival biopsy	WBC ↑↑ Abnormal platelets Hb urea

N. = normal, E.T. = Essential thrombocytopenia..

	Haemphilia A	VWD
Platelets	N.	N.
B.T.	N.	(↑)
PT	N.	N.
PTT	(↑)	(↑)
Other I_x	↓ Factor VIII ↓ VWF	↓ Factor VIII ↓↓ VWF

Vitamin K deficiency: PT → (↑↑), PTT → ↑, platelets → N., B.T → N.

Liver diseases & DIC: ALL I_x → ABNORMAL

Trick: Pancytopenia = ↓↓ platelets, ↓↓ WBC, ↓↓ Hb. → For example, in aplastic anemia, leukemia & Kala-azar..

5- PEDIATRICS — FOLLOW UP CHARTS..

Follow up charts:

Patient with meningitis:

General examination (especially the consciousness & posture)..
Vital signs..
Fontanelle, OFC, pupil & fundoscopy..
Cranial nn. examination (especially the 6th)..
Meningeal signs..
Upper & lower limbs neurological examination..
Input & output fluid & weight..
Any new investigation should be checked..

Patient with nephrotic syndrome:

Edema..
Urine output..
Weight..
Vital signs..
General wellbeing..
Steroid S.E..
Any complication (infection, thrombosis & hyperlipidemia)..
G.U.E & serum albumin..

Patient with Guillain Barré syndrome:

General examination..
Vital signs..
Upper & lower limbs neurological examination..
Cranial nn. Examination (especially the 6th)..
History of chocking or regurgitation..
Assessment for bulbar involvement..
Reflexes & autonomic dysfunction (such as profuse sweating, palpitation & postural hypotension)
Sphincter disturbances..

Diabetes mellitus:

Name, age, date & time
Body weight & surface area..
Pulse rate & B.P..
PH, RBS, S. electrolytes, insulin dose..
Fluid input, output & signs of cerebral edema..
Any other notes..

5- PEDIATRICS
DEVELOPMENT MADE VERY EASY ' by Dr. M.O.M '..

Developmental milestones:

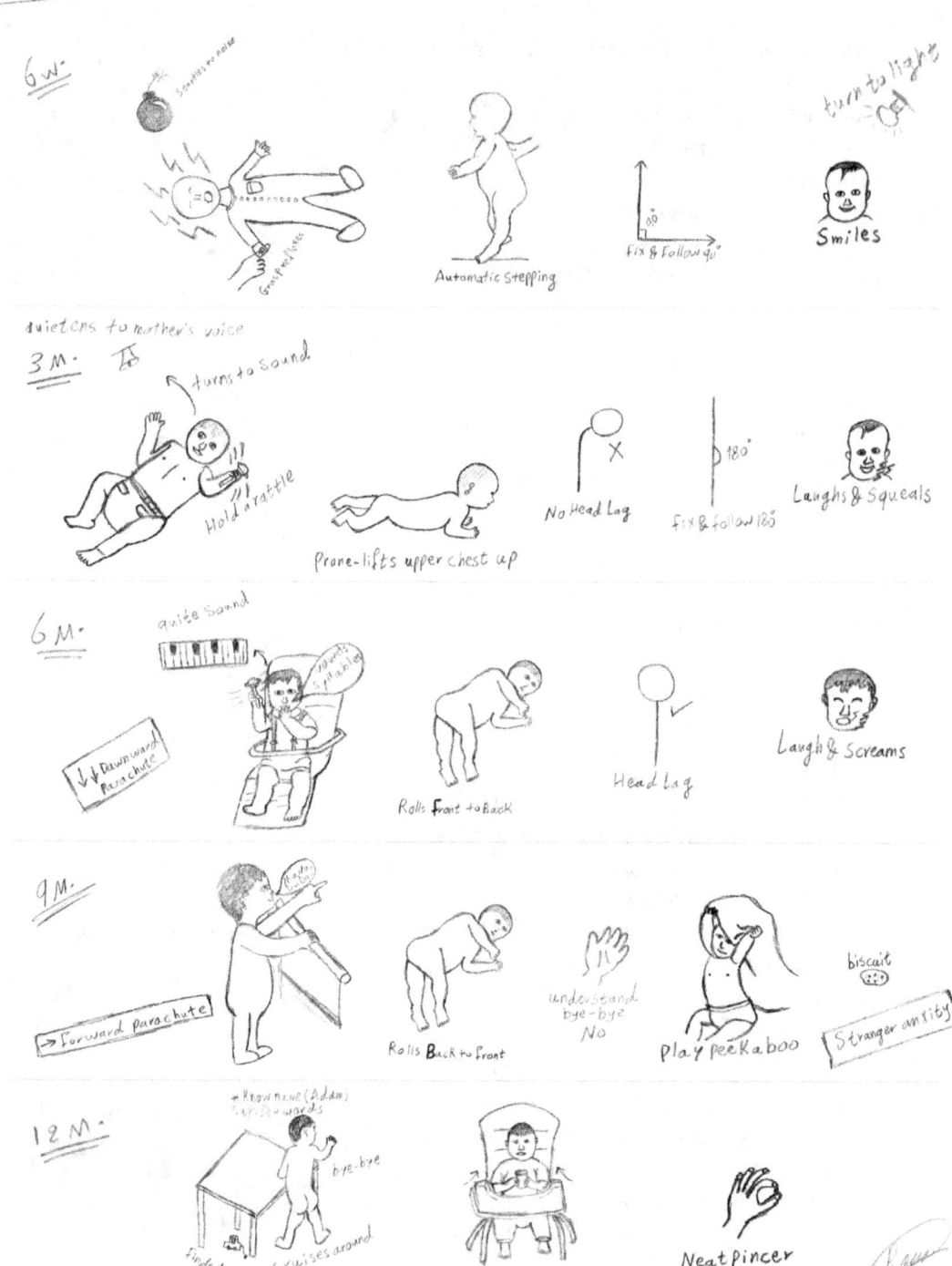

5- PEDIATRICS
DEVELOPMENT MADE VERY EASY ' by Dr. M.O.M '..

15 M:

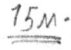
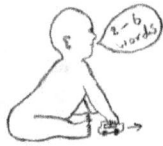
Broad Based Gait

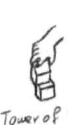
Tower of 2 Bricks

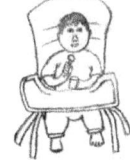
Uses cup & spoon

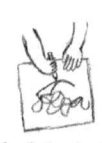
To & Fro Scribble

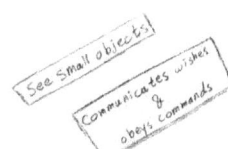
See small objects
Communicates wishes & obeys commands

18 M:

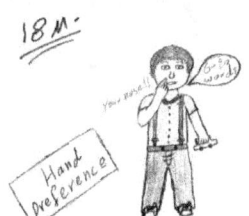
Hand Preference

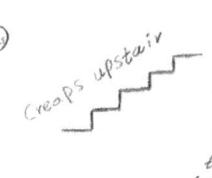
Creeps upstair

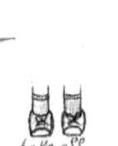
Take off socks & shoes

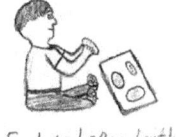
Feed independently

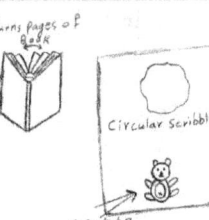
Turns pages of book
Circular Scribble
Point to picture

2 y:

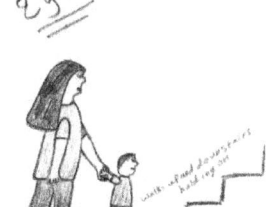
walks up and down stairs holding on

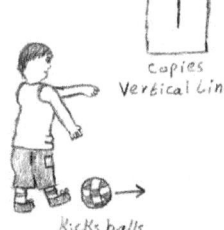
Kicks balls

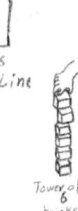
Copies Vertical Line

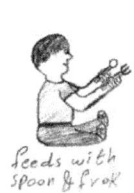
Tower of 6 bricks

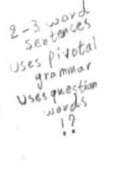
Feeds with spoon & fork

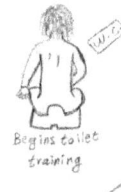
Begins toilet training

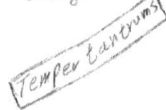
2-3 word sentences
Uses pivotal grammar
Uses question words !?

Temper tantrums

3 y:

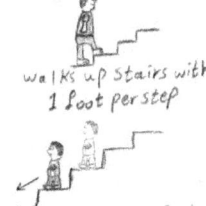
walks up stairs with 1 foot per step

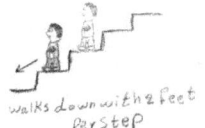
walks down with 2 feet per step

Tip-Toe

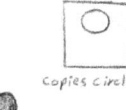
Copies circle

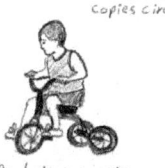
Pedals tricycle

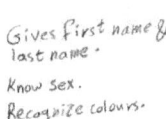
Gives first name & last name.
Know sex.
Recognize colours.

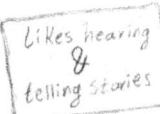
Likes hearing & telling stories

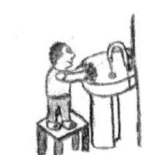
Washes hands and brushes teeth
eats with fork & spoon

4 y:

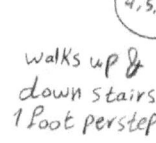
walks up & down stairs 1 foot per step

Hops

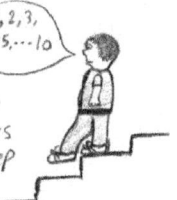
Copies cross
Draw man

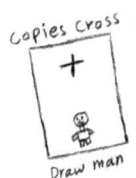

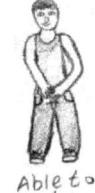
Able to undress

5 y:

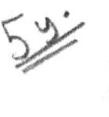
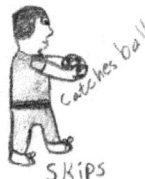
Catches ball
Skips

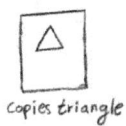
Copies triangle

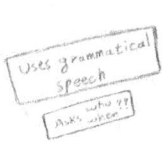
Uses grammatical speech
Asks who ??
Asks when

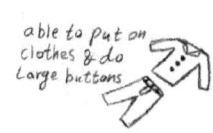
able to put on clothes & do large buttons

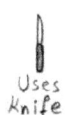
Uses knife

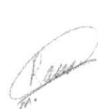

5- PEDIATRICS — DRUGS ' ESSENTIALS NOTES '..

DRUGS ' ESSENTIALS NOTES ' :

Diazepam amp. (Valium) :

Indication : In stop convulsions
(Not to treat it .. So, it is used in E.R. not at home)

Main S/E : Respiratory depression
(So, monitor the respiratory rate)

Dose : 0.1 – 0.3 mg/kg/dose , Given by slow diluted I.V.
(If there is no I.V. access , you can give it rectally)
Can be repeated 3 times in status epilepticus

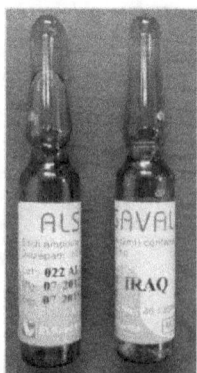

Phenytoin (Epanutin) amp. & Phenobarbital (Luminal) amp. :

Indication : In status epilepticus (2nd line of Rx)
In convulsion (Whatever the cause)
Head trauma
Subarachnoid hemorrhage

Main S/E : Change in the level of consciousness
Nausea & vomiting

Dose : Loading dose 15 – 20 mg/kg/dose   I.V. slow infusion
Maintenance dose 5 mg/kg in 2 divided doses   I.V. slow infusion

Compatible with N/S , never give it with G/W

Note : Whenever patient more than 6 years comes with fever , photophobia & convulsion .. this is unlikely to be febrile convulsion because age of febrile convulsion is (5 months – 6 months)

Note : Phenytoin → When we need to remain the patient conscious (ex. Meningitis)
Phenobarbital → When sedation is needed (Cerebral palsy & hypoglycemic fit)

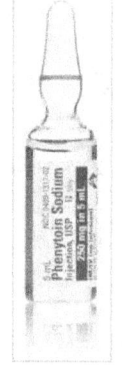 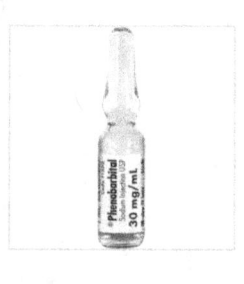

Hydrocortisone Vial & Dexamethasone amp (Decadron amp.):

Action: H.C. is more rapid (So, used in acute stage like *Asthma & Anaphylaxis*)
Dexamethasone is more potent & longer duration

Main S/E : Hypertension
Hyperglycemia
Gastric upset
Paresthesia (For Decadron)

Dose : H.C. → 10 mg/kg/day I.V. (Can be repeated)
either Once (10 mg/kg),
Twice (5 then 5 mg/kg) or
Thrice (3 , 3 then 3 mg/kg)

Dexamethasone → 0.1 – 0.3 mg/kg in 4 divided doses I.V.
0.6 mg/kg/dose I.V.
(Used in meningitis to decrease cerebral edema)

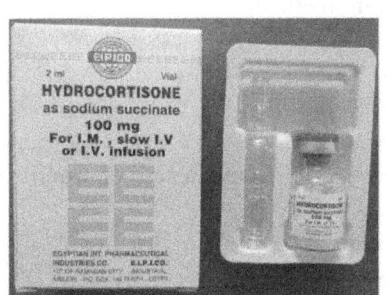
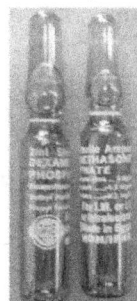

Sodium Bicarbonate NaHCO₃ 8.4% (and there is 7% & 9.5%) amp. :

Indication : In severe acidosis such as DKA &
Renal failure *(When PH is less than 7.2)*

Main S/E : Hypokalemia
Hypoglycemia
Cerebral edema

Dose : 1cc/kg/dose *4 times daily* I.V. slow
(But not more than 25 mg/dose)

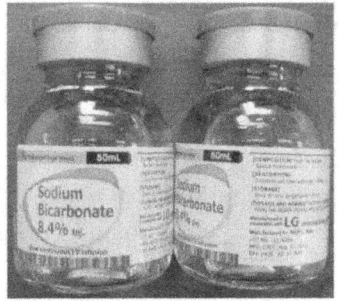

5- PEDIATRICS : DRUGS ' ESSENTIALS NOTES '..

Metoclopramide (Plasil) amp. :

Note : It is dopamine antagonist

Indication : For nausea & vomiting

Main S/E : Oculogyric crises
   (So, it is used with caution in pediatric & treated with *Allermin* & Atropine)

Dose : 0.1-0.2 mg/kg/dose I.V. or I.M.

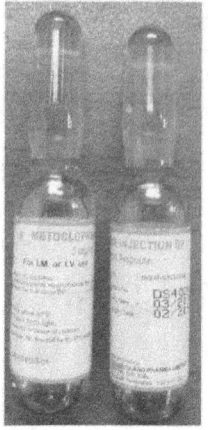

Epinephrine (Adrenaline) amp. :

Note : It is sympathomimetic drug

Indication : Anaphylaxis (given S.C.)
   Cardiac standstill (I.V. or Intracardiac)
   Anaphylactic shock as (S.C.)
   Sever laryngeal edema in case of croup

Main S/E : Tachycardia
   Hypertension

Dose : 0.01 mg/kg/dose

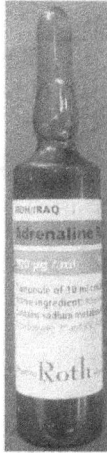

Aminophylline amp. :

Indication : : In severe asthma not responding to salbutamol & H.C. as bronchodilator

Main S/E : Tachycardia
   Dysrhythmia
   Nausea & Vomiting

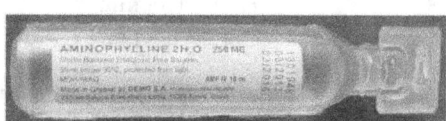

Dose : 3-5 mg/kg continuous I.V. slow infusion in 30 cc G/W 5% over 1/2 h
   or 3 times bolus 5 mg/kg/hr

5- PEDIATRICS — DRUGS ' ESSENTIALS NOTES '..

Furosemide (Lasix) amp. :

Note : It is loop diuretics

Indication : In fluid overload including
- Over-replacement in treatment of dehydration
- Edema
- Hypertension

Main S/E : Hypovolemia
- Hypocalcaemia
- Hypokalemia
- Hyperuricemia

Dose : 1-2 mg/kg/dose I.V. *(Can be repeated 3 times)*

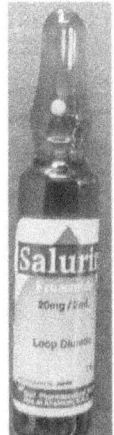

Tranexamic acid (Cyklokapron) amp. :

Note : Antifibrinolytic agent

Indication : In mucosal bleeding *(gum , nasal , GIT , vaginal , uterine .. etc.)*

Main S/E : Thrombosis
- Hypotension
- Nausea & Vomiting

C.I. : In case of hematuria
(Because it may cause obstructive uropathy & acute renal failure)

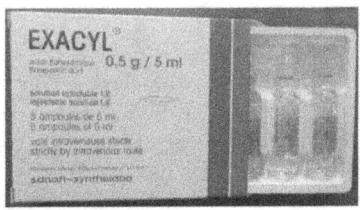

Dose : 45 mg/kg /day in 3 divided doses slow I.V. infusion with N/S

Hyosine-N-Butylbromide (Buscopan) amp. :

Note : Anticholinergic drug

Indication : In acute spasm of bowel
(Colicky abdominal pain)

Main S/E : Lazy bowel syndrome
- Paralytic ileus

Dose : 0.1 – 0.2 mg/kg/dose I.V.

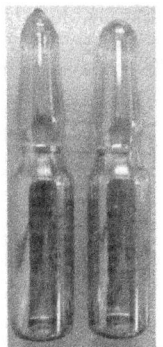

5- PEDIATRICS — DRUGS ' ESSENTIALS NOTES '..

Vit. K ' Phytomenadione ' amp. :

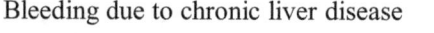

Indication : To decrease the risk of bleeding in neonate after birth *(hemorrhagic disease of new born at day 2-7 of life)*

Bleeding due to chronic liver disease

Dose : Therapeutic → 5 mg/day single dose daily until the bleeding stops
Prophylactic → 1 mg/day
I.M. or I.V

In liver disease is given in alternate days with plasma

Salbutamol (Ventolin solution) :

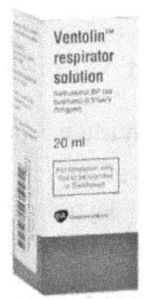
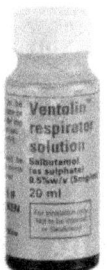

Indication : In acute bronchospasm
(it is act on smooth muscle of bronchus causing relaxation)

Main S/E : Tachycardia
Tremor

Dose : 0.6 mg/kg in 24 hr
Ventolin nebulizer → *Add 0.5 cc Salbutamol solution in 1.5 cc N/S & put it in nebulizer (can repeat it 3 times)*

Ranitidin amp. (Zantac) & Cimetidine amp. (Tagamet):

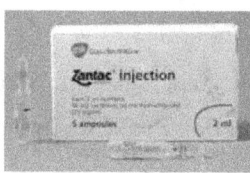

Note : It is H$_2$ blocker

Indication : Gastric ulcer
GERD
Stress ulcer
Esophageal varices

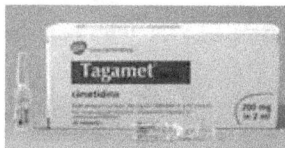

Dose : Ranitidin 1-2 mg/kg/dose I.V. X 2
Cimetidine 10 mg/kg/dose I.V. X 2

5- PEDIATRICS — DRUGS ' ESSENTIALS NOTES '..

Sodium stibogluconate (Pentostam) :

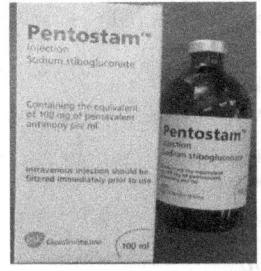
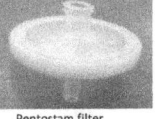

Pentostam filter

Indication : Anti-leishmaniasis

Main S/E : Nausea & vomiting
Abdominal pain
Elevated liver enzymes
Fever
ECG changes

Dose : 20 mg/kg/day once daily for 20 days
I.M. or *I.V. infusion with filter*

Potassium (Kcl) amp. :

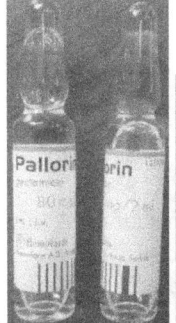

Indication : For treatment of Hypokalemia
DKA
Dehydration with repeated vomiting
Paralytic ileus

Dose : 1 ml/kg
Each ml (cc) = 2 meq Kcl
So, each kg needs 1 cc .. For example, we have 10 kg infant who needs 1000 cc fluid , we add 10 ccs Kcl to 1000 cc fluid (2 pints) but never put more than 10 cc of Kcl in one liter .. *(So, do not exceeds 5 cc / pint of fluid)*

Gentamicin amp. & Amikacin amp. :

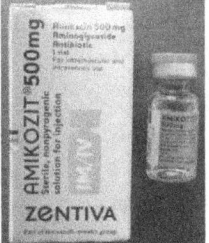

Note : It is antibiotic (Aminoglycoside group) ..
Strong against G-ve and may use for G+ve

Indication : UTI
Gastroenteritis

Dose : Gentamicin amp 3-5 mg/kg/day 2 divided doses
Amikacin amp 15 mg/kg/day in 2 divided doses
I.M. or I.V.

Cefotaxime (Claforan) , Ceftriaxone (Rocephin) , Ceftazidime (Fortum) Vial :

Note : There are Cephalosporins group of ABTs

All have the same efficacy on Gram +ve microorganisms *but there efficacy on Gram –ve increase respectively (Fortum > Rocephin > Claforan)*

Ceftazidim is a potent anti-pseudomonal ABT

Dose :

Claforan 100 mg/kg/day in 2 divided doses

Ceftriaxone 50-100 mg/kg/day in 2 divided doses

Dose : I.M. or I.V. infusion

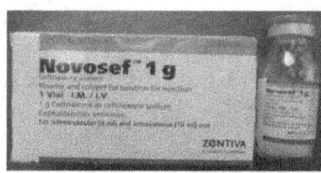

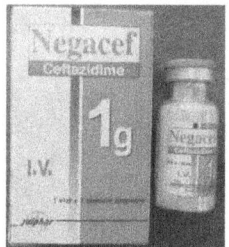 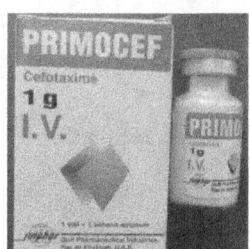

Calcium Gluconate 10% amp. :

Indication : Hypocalcaemia
Hyperkalemia *(To protect the heart)*
Renal failure

Dose : 1 cc/kg/day by I.V. infusion in G/W per 6 hrs

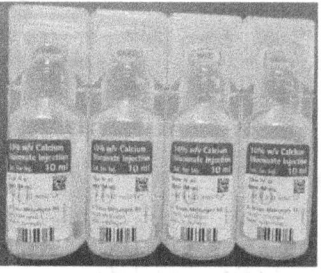

Chlorpheniramine (Allermine) amp. :

Note : Antihistamine

Dose : 1 mg/kg/dose I.M. or I.V.

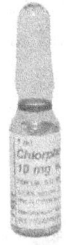

5- PEDIATRICS — DRUGS ' ESSENTIALS NOTES '..

Atropine amp. :

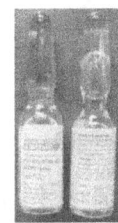

Indication : For Bradycardia caused by Organophosphorus poisoning

Dose : 0.01 mg/kg I.V.

Ampiclox vial :

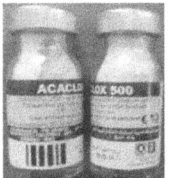

Note : It is Ampicillin and Cloxacillin

C.I. : in Penicillin allergy

Dose : 200 mg/kg/day in 4 divided doses I.M or I.V.

Metronidazole (Flagyl) bottle :

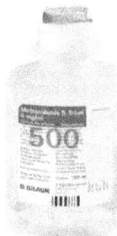

Indication : For Anaerobes & Parasites

Dose : 5-7 mg/kg/dose X 3
      (1.5 cc/kg/dose X 3) I.V.

Acetaminophen (Antipyrol) syrup :

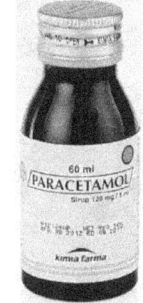

Indication : For pain & fever relief

Dose : 10-15 mg/kg/dose X 3 oral

Digoxen amp. :

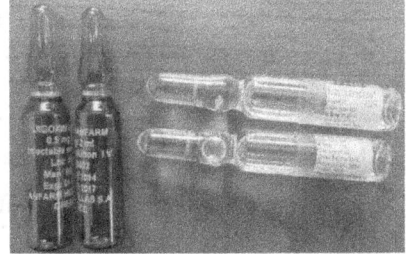

Digitalization : 0.02 – 0.04 mg/kg/dose
              1/2 dose → (1st) 8 hr.
              1/4 dose → (2nd) 8 hr.
              1/4 dose → (3rd) 8 hr.

Maintenance : 0.005 – 0.01 mg/kg/day
            (LAST DOSE / 2)

5- PEDIATRICS : DRUGS ' ESSENTIALS NOTES '..

INSULIN vial :

Soluble :

, clear solution

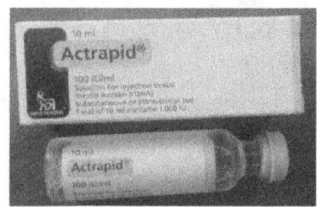

Lente:

LIGHT BLUE or GREEN vial, cloudy

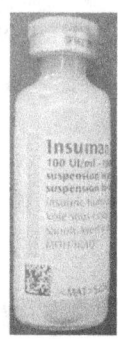

Mixed:

Brown vial, cloudy , written on it 30 \ 70 (30% soluble + 70% Lente)

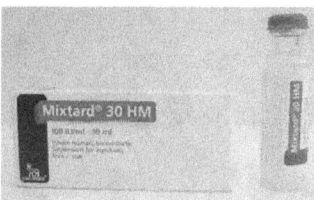

GLUCAGON vial :

Indication : For severe hypoglycemic reactions in patients with D.M. treated with insulin

Dose : < 20 kg : 0.5 mg subcutaneous , IM or IV
> 20 kg : 1 mg subcutaneous , IM or IV

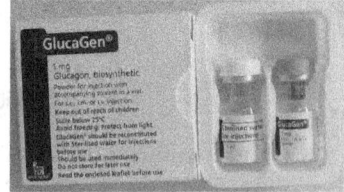

INTRAVENOUS FLUIDS ' ESSENTIALS NOTES ' :

Saline :

Note : Isotonic , contains no glucose

Indication : Use for replacement of deficit in treatment of severe dehydration
As *20 cc / Kg / 1hr* N/S (Shoot)

Components : Normal saline 0.9 % (N/S) → Na^+ =150 meq/L + Cl^- =150 meq/L
Ringer's lactate (R/L) → Na^+ =130 meq/L + Cl^- =110 meq/L
K^+ *=5 meq/L* + Ca^{++} *=2 meq/L*

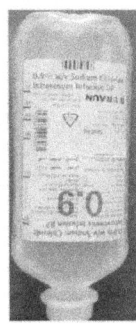
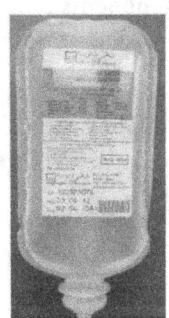

Glucose water (G/W) :

Indication : For treatment of hypoglycemic state such in
diabetic hypoglycemia
in liver disease

Different concentrations available :
G/W 5% → 5 gm glucose / 100 cc water
G/W 10% → 10 gm glucose / 100 cc water
G/W 50% → 50 gm glucose / 100 cc water

Note : 1 pint of 5% G/W → is 500 cc → so, contains 25 gm glucose
1 pint of 10% G/W → is 500 cc → so, contains 50 gm glucose
1 vial of 50% G/W (Hypertonic) → is 20 cc → so, contains 10 gm glucose

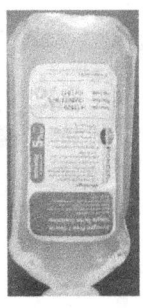
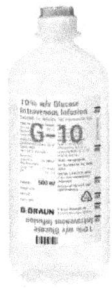
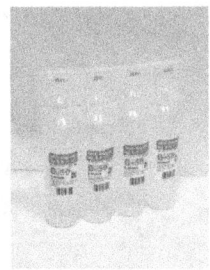

Glucose Saline (G/S):

Indication : For maintenance fluid requirement

1/5 G/S Maintenance :
- 1st 10 Kg → 100 cc / Kg
- 2nd 10 Kg → 50 cc / Kg
- > 20 Kg → 20 cc / Kg

Components :

1/5 Glucose Saline (G/S) → Na^+ = 30 meq/L + Cl^- = 30 meq/L
        Glucose = 40 gram/L

1/2 Glucose Saline (G/S) → Na^+ = 75 meq/L + Cl^- = 75 meq/L
        Glucose = 50 gram/L

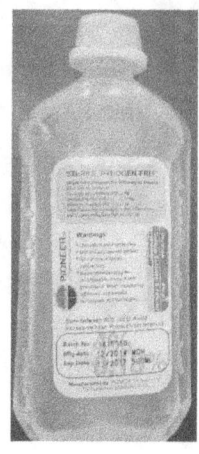

5- PEDIATRICS : BLOOD PRODUCTS ' ESSENTIALS NOTES '..

Blood products ' ESSENTIALS NOTES ' :

Whole blood :

Indication : Exchange transfusion
Replacement of blood loss as hypovolemia , shock , bleeding .. etc.

Calculation : 20 cc/kg

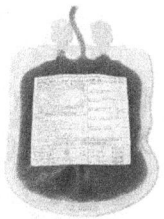

Packed Red Blood Cells (PRBC) :

Indication : Anemia , Fluid overload , H.F. , Chronic blood loss

Calculation : 10 cc/kg

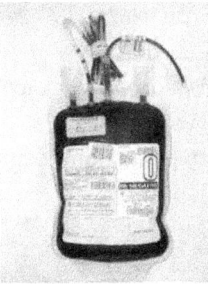

Plasma :

Indication : Bleeding varices

Calculation : 15 cc/kg

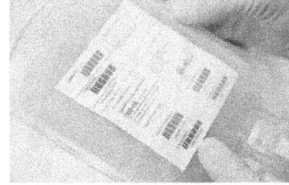

Platelets :

Indication : Thrombocytopenia

Calculation : 1 pint / 5kg

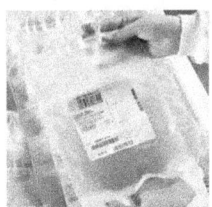

5- PEDIATRICS — OTHER IMPORTANT TOPICS..

Lumbar puncture:

Indication:

Diagnostic: suspected meningitis or G.B.S..
Therapeutic: drug administration,
  spinal anesthesia,
  decompression of spinal fluid to ↓↓ I.C.P..

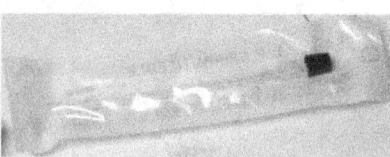
By my colleague's camera..

Contraindication:

Bleeding tendency (relative), infection at the site of insertion, compromised cardiopulmonary status, & signs of ↑↑ I.C.P. in > 2 years old child (anterior fontanelle closed)..

Complication:

Local infection..
Trauma..
Bleeding..
Headache, backache..
Herniation..
Implantation of epidural tumor..

Bone marrow aspiration & biopsy:

Indication:

Suspicion of malignancy..
Unexplained hepatosplenomegaly..
Fever of unknown origin..
I.T.P.
Anemia of unknown cause..

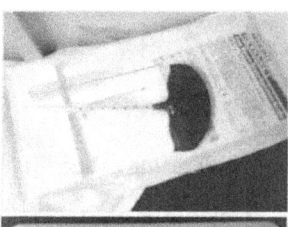
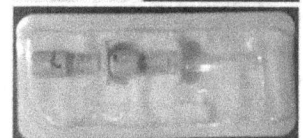
By my colleague's camera..

Contraindication:

Bleeding tendency..
Hypertension..
Compromises cardiopulmonary status (*unstable for G.A.*)..

Complication:

Local infection..
Trauma..

Exchange transfusion:

Indication:

For *indirect* hyperbilirubinemia..

The total amount of blood exchanged:

= Weight X 85 ml X 2

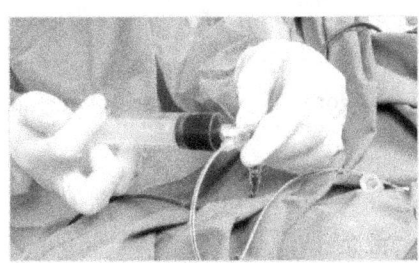

Complication:

Acute:
Hypoglycemia..
Hypoxia & acidosis..
Transient bradycardia with or without hypocalcaemia..
Hypocalcaemia..
Thrombosis..
Apnea with bradycardia..
Necrotizing enterocolitis (rare)..
Infection: C.M.V., H.I.V..
Death..

Late:
Cholestasis..
Anemia (late)..
Mild graft versus host disease..
Inspissated bile syndrome (rare)..
Portal vein thrombosis & portal hypertension..

Name of umbilical vein catheter:

Is a polyvinyl catheter..

NOTES:

- Exchange transfusion is carried out over 45 – 60 min with alternating aspiration & infusion of 20 ml of blood (each time)..

- A calcium infusion (1-2 ml/kg of 10% calcium gluconate given slowly via a central line) may be required to correct hypocalcaemia.

5- PEDIATRICS — OTHER IMPORTANT TOPICS..

Phototherapy:

Indication:

For *indirect* hyperbilirubinemia..

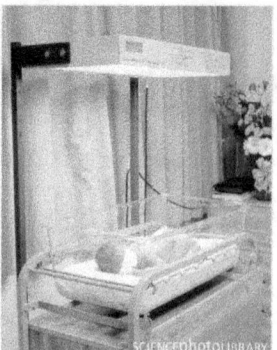

Complication:

Over heating & dehydration..
Loose stool & diarrhea..
Chilling..
Eye injury & nasal closure (uncommon)..
Bronze baby syndrome..
Erythmatous maculopapular rash & purpuric rash with transient porphyria..

Contraindication:

Direct hyperbilirubinemia..
Porphyria..

NOTES:

- By using high intensity light, in the blue range 420 – 470 nm..

- The therapeutic effect of phototherapy depends on: wavelength of light, distance, amount of skin exposed & the presence of hemolysis..

- Light source distance from the infant is 45 cm, the infant should be naked except for eye patches & the baby should be turned frequently every 2 hours for maximum exposure..

- **Intensive Phototherapy:** used when indirect bilirubin reaches maximum level that needs exchange, so by using special light & the use of fiber optic phothearapy blanket under the baby for maximum exposure (430-490 nm wavelength)

Ventolin nubulizer (Salbutamol):

- You should educate the family about the ventolin nubulizer..
- Take 0.5 cc of ventolin then add 1.5 cc of normal saline to it..
- Put it in the nubulizer and use it over 10 – 15 minutes..
- Can repeat it 3 times only because of its side effects..

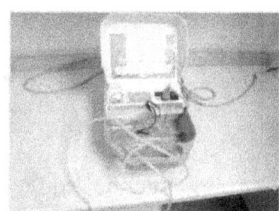

By my colleague's camera..

Indication: Asthma..

S.E.:

Tremor..
Tachycardia & arrhythmia..
Repeated vomiting..

5- PEDIATRICS — OTHER IMPORTANT TOPICS..

Different types of drips:

Trick: Small – with NO filter

Large..

Small – with filter for blood clots

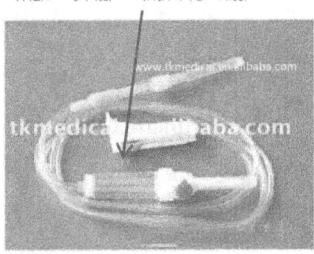
I.V. macrodrip (15 drops = 1 ml)..

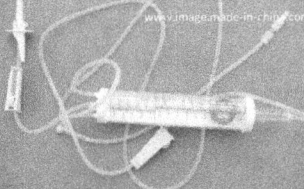
Microdrip.. (Burette-Transfusion-Set)

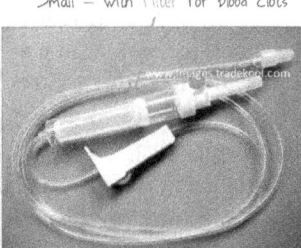
Blood transfusion macrodrip..

Microdrip (Burette-Transfusion-Set):

60 drops = 1 ml

Uses: To give small amount of fluid..
To give some drugs (like ciprofloxacin)..
To give specific electrolytes (like Ca^{+2} in 1 hour & $NaHCO_3$ in 20 min.)
BUT NOT K^+..

We close it by a simple lock to prevent any infection..

Intraosseous needle:

Indication:

Difficulty in establishing venous access:
in burns, obesity, edema or seizures.
Necessity for rapid high volumes fluid infusion:
in hypovolemic shock & burns.
Access to systemic venous circulation:
in cardiopulmonary arrest, burns, medication infusion..etc

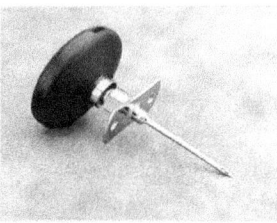

Contraindication:

- Infection or burn at entry site   - Osteopenia or osteopetrosis   - Osteogenesis imperfecta
- Ipsilateral fracture of extremity   - Unable to locate the landmark
- Previous attempt at the same site or diffirent location in the same bone

Complication:

Infection, extravasations of blood or infusion, compartment syndrome, bent needle or bone fracture ..etc

Positioning:

- Proximal tibia, distal to the tibial tuberosity..   - Distal end of the radial bone..
- Proximal metaphysic of the humerus..   - Distal tibia proximal to the medial malleolus..
- Distal femur, above the femur plateau..   - Sternum..   - Calcaneus..

5- PEDIATRICS — OTHER IMPORTANT TOPICS..

Liver biopsy:

Indication:

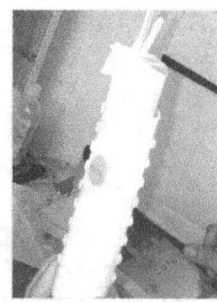
By my colleague's camera..

- Investigation of suspected diffuse liver disease, such as infective, autoimmune, cholestatic and congenital forms of hepatitis, metabolic liver disease, such as Wilson's disease ..etc
- Investigation of focal liver disease, such as, teratoma, mesenchymal hamartoma, hepatoblastoma, rhabdoid tumour.. etc.
- Management of liver transplant..
- Management of drug therapies that affect the liver parenchyma..

Contraindication:

- A patient who is too unstable or critically unwell to undergo this procedure..
- Significant coagulopathy..
- Significant thrombocytopaenia..
- Significant ascites..

Complication:

Intraperitoneal haemorrhage, biliary peritonitis, haemobilia and injury to the duodenum, colon or lung. The risk of significant bleeding after an image-guided percutaneous liver biopsy..

Urine analysis (urine dipstick):

Instructions:

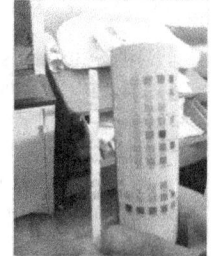
By my colleague's camera..

- All samples should be midstream and collected in a clean sterile container..
- Suprapubic aspiration or fresh catheter samples are ideal, but not always practical..
- Immerse the dipstick completely in fresh urine and withdraw immediately, drawing edge along rim of container to remove excess..
- Hold dipstick horizontally before reading..

For: Color, Turbidity, Odor, Specific gravity, pH, Haematuria, Proteinuria, Glucose, Ketones, Bilirubin & Urobilinogen test, Leucocyte esterase & Urobilinogen..

Other important topics:

You *have to* know something about:
- Fluid,
- Blood products,
- Drugs in pediatrics..

CHAPTER 6

GYNECOLOGY & OBSTETRICS

Contents:

H$_x$ CASE SHEET	196
EXAMINATION	
Obstetric abdominal E$_x$	200
Gynecological P.V. E$_x$	202
Clinical pelvimetry	203
Post operative assessment	204
PARTOGRAM	205
FORCEPS & INSTRUMENTS	212
OXYTOCIN & METHERGINE	223

6- GYNE. & OBSTETRICS   HISTORY TAKING [CASE SHEET]..

HISTORY CASE SHEET :

DEMOGRAPHY DATA:
> Triple name :
> Age :
> Occupation :
> Residence :
> Blood group & Rh : For the patient & her husband ..
> Consanguinity :

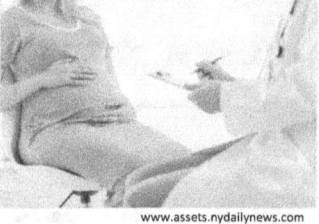

> Date of admission :
> Date of taking H_x :

> **Gravida (G) :**
> *No. of pregnancy including this one (regardless the outcome & weeks of gestation)*

> **Para (P) :**
> *Deliveries after 28 w. of gestation*

> **Abortion (A) :**
> *Fetal death before 20 wks. of gestation (cause ? , curettage ?)*

> **Last Menstrual Period (LMP) :** *Day / Month / Year*

> **Expected day of delivery (EDD) :** *We add 7 days & 9 months (or -3 months) to LMP*

>> *If No. of months of LMP is 1 , 2 or 3 , we add 9 months to get EDD*
>> *If No. of months of LMP is 4 , 5 , 6 , …… 12 we subtract 3 months to get EDD*
>> *Don't forget to increase the No. of year (e.g. 2013 → 2014)*

> **Gestational age (GA) :** *Either counts from 1st day of LMP (add 1 week for every 3 months) or*
> *From EDD (40 w.) subtract till reach present date*

CHIEF COMPLAINT & DURATION:
> ex. Vaginal bleeding of 7 days duration

Hx OF PRESENT ILLNESS:
> Mention the details of patient's condition
> Mention the details of :
>> 1st Trimester (1-14 w.)..
>> 2nd Trimester (14-28 w.)..
>> 3rd Trimester (28 -42 w.)..

1st Trimester (1-14 wks.) :

Nausea , Vomiting ? *(due to increase B-HCG level)*
Appetite ?
Fatigue ? *(due to anemia)*
Backache ?
Any swelling in the body ?
ANC (antenatal care) ?
Early vaginal bleeding ?
Burning micturition ?
Color of urine ?
Taking any drugs ?
Constipation ?
X-ray exposure ? *(Teratogenic effect)*
Any trauma or disease ?

2nd Trimester (14-28 wks.) :

Quickening (first fetus movement) : *Primi-gravida between (18-20 wks.)*
                                       Multi-gravida between (16-18 wks.)
Weight gain ? , Any swelling in the body ? *(Due to fluid retention)*
Appetite ?
Vomiting ?
Constipation ?
Increase in urine amount ?
Frequent micturition ?
Palpitation ? *(Due to anemia)*
Tingling ? , numbness ?
Vision ?

3rd Trimester (28 -42 wks.) :

Fetal movement ?
Headache ? , Tingling ? , Numbness ? , Fit ? *(Eclampsia ??)*
Any vaginal discharge ? , *Show* ? *(Bloody cervical mucus indicate cervical dilatation)*
Any leg swelling?
Palpitation ?
H_x of anemia ?
Shortness of breath ?
Chest pain ?

IN ANY vaginal bleeding , Ask about :

Amount ? , *Any clots ? (it means large amount)*
Painful ?
Associated with cycle ? ,
First time ?
Any other site ? , Any medical illness ?
Any drugs ? , Any family H_x ?

6- GYNE. & OBSTETRICS — HISTORY TAKING [CASE SHEET]..

SYSTEMS REVIEW:
(In case of +ve finding , You have to ask further questions to get more details ..)
(The details was mentioned in CHAPTER 1 ..)

PAST OBSTETRICAL Hx :

When get married ?
When get the 1st pregnancy ? (Any period of infertility ? , Contraceptive method ?)
Duration between 1st & 2nd pregnancy ? , contraception method ?
Hx of each pregnancy :
    No. of pregnancy ? Pass smoothly , Any complications (Bleeding , Infections ,
                        Fit , Vomiting , D.M. or H.T.) ?
    Duration ?
    A.N.C .. Regular ?
    No. of children ? , Gender ? , H_x of death ? , *Term , pre- or post- term ?*
    Delivered by normal vaginal delivery or c/s (Type)?
    Spontaneous or induced (Onset) ?
    At hospital or home (Place) ?
    When (Date) ?
    With any complications (PPH , Puerperium , Sepsis .. etc.) ?
    Weight, Crying time & Feeding of the baby ?
    Normal or abnormal baby ? (Any congenital anomalies or neonatal jaundice ?)

    Puerperium : Duration of staying in the bed ?
            Prolong vaginal discharge after delivery (Lochia) ?
            Any leg swelling (D.V.T.) ?
            Any bleeding ?
            Any other problem (U.T.I., Incontinence , fever , Rigor ,Mastitis
                      , Urine retention , .. etc.) ?

PAST GYNECOLOGICAL H..

Date of 1st cycle (Menarche) ?
Periods : *Duration ? , Regular or irregular ? , Frequency ?, Painful ?*
Any pelvic pain ? *(Pain analysis)*
Any vaginal discharge ? (color ? , odor ? , amount ?)
Last pap smear ?
If she is present after menopause .. so, at what age ?
Any H_x of bleeding ? , Post coital bleeding ?
Any H_x of hospitalization or blood transfusion ? , Curettage , Cautery or Operation ?
Any gynecological problem ?
Any period of infertility (Time , Frequency of intercourse , Any pain or sex difficulties) ?
Contraception ? *(In details)* , Drug intake ?

PAST-MEDICAL Hx :

Hypertension ? , D.M. ? , Asthma ? , Rubella ? ... etc.
(In case of +ve finding ask about Time ,Onset , Duration , Treated or not .. etc.)
Any admission to the hospital & the cause ?

PAST-SURGICAL Hx :

Any previous surgery ? When ? , Type ? , Any complications ?
H_x of blood transfusion ?

DRUG Hx :

Any drug allergy ?
Any chronic use of drug ?

FAMILY Hx :

Any H_x of familial H.T. , D.M. , Bleeding disorder or Mental retardation ?

SOCIO-ECONOMIC Hx :

Marital state : (Married , Separated , Divorced or Widow) ?
Smoking ?
Alcohol ?
Housing condition ?
Drug addict ?

6- GYNE. & OBSTETRICS   EXAMINATION..

Obstetric abdominal examination:

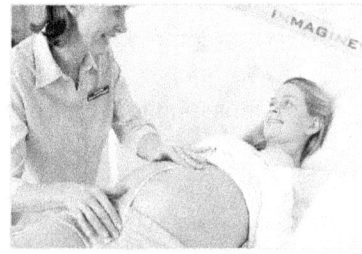
www.images.inmagine.com

First: greet the patient,
introduce yourself,
take permission for examination,
explain to the patient what you will do,
hand washing,
make sure patient privacy,
good exposure ' *from above the nipple to the mid-thigh* '..

Inspection: assess the uterus (symmetry), any scar, stria, linea nigra, distended veins,
umbilicus, movement with respiration (*limited*),
fetal movement & hair distribution..

Trick: to see the symmetry, you have to go in front of patient at the foot end of the bed..

Palpation: ' *rub your hands, knee sitting, ask if he has any pain.., see to the face of the patient* '..

Superficial: all 9 quadrants for mass or tenderness..

Deep: **Symphysis-fundal height** → feel the xiphisternum, localize the fundus, put the tape measure (the centimeters degrees face to the abdomen), feel the pubic symphysis then measure the S.F.H..

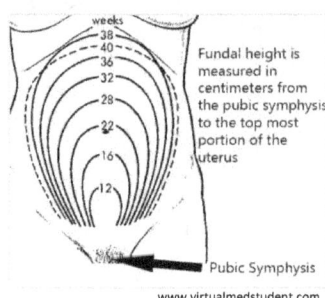
www.virtualmedstudent.com

Fundal grip → (*look to the patient face & use all your palms not only the fingers*)..
breach (large, soft, irregular& there is no groove with the back),
head (small, hard, globular, there is a groove between it & the back)..

Lateral grip → poles (*single or multiple*), lie & altitude, position & the liquor..
back (firm, smooth & convex) & the poles (knobby & mobile)..

Pelvic grip → 2 maneuver (engagement & the role of 5th) & the presentation ?

Then → Liver: at the right lateral border of uterus & ascend..
Spleen: at the left lateral border of uterus & ascend..
Kidneys: as usual, but it is difficult..

6- GYNE. & OBSTETRICS EXAMINATION..

Percussion: usually not done *'because, it is traumatic '..*

Auscultation: bowel sounds,
    fetal heart rate
    & renal bruit (from the back at the site of costophrenic angle)..

Don't forget to mention: P.V., inguinal & perineal region examination & P.R. examination..

At the end: cover the patient & thank her..

After you complete the examination:

You have to summarize the following:

Fundal height (the gestational age)..

Lie (longitudinal or oblique)..

Presentation..

Position (Where is the back of the baby !!)..

Level of engagement..

Altitude (usually in flexion)..

Single or multiple..
Amount of liquor..
   polyhydramnios → large for date, ballotable with transmitted thrill,
   oligohydramnios → fetal part easily palpated..

Uterine consistency..
Uterine contraction..

6- GYNE. & OBSTETRICS EXAMINATION..

Gynecological P.V. examination:

First: greet the patient,
introduce yourself,
verbal consent [presence of one of her relative],
explain to the patient what you will do,
hand washing & wear gloves,
make sure patient privacy,
proper position (flexion of the hips & knees)..
good exposure..
cleaning with antiseptic..

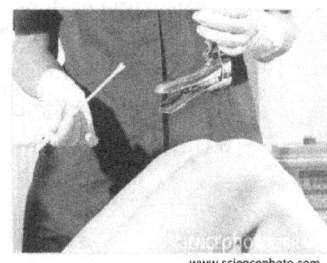

Inspection: Hair distribution, clitoris, ulcer, redness, mass, scar or discharge..
Ask her to cough (for incontinence) & strain (for prolapsed)..
Then (separate the labia majora by left hand with 2 fingers)..
Introduce the speculum (*don't forget to put a lubricant*) to see the cervix, lateral wall of vagina & perform pap smear..

Palpation: *' don't forget to put a lubricant '*..
One finger → vaginal wall, adnexal tenderness & cervical excitation..
Two finger → (bimanual examination)
size, mobility, tenderness & consistency of uterus, retroverted or anteverted uterus, adnexal mass & tenderness, pouch of douglas (posteriorly)..

Remove your fingers..
Clean the area..

Don't forget to mention: P.R. examination..

At the end: cover the patient & thank her..

Clinical pelvimetry:

Inlet: Normally, you can't reach the promontory of sacrum..
But, if you can → this is the **diagonal** conjugate..
(**diagonal** - 1.5 cm) = *true conjugate*..

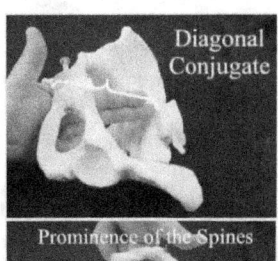

Cavity: Palpate the anterior surface of the sacrum (from above downward) → straight or concave ' *normally, it is concave* '..

Ischial spines → (prominent, diverted or inverted) & the interspinous distance..

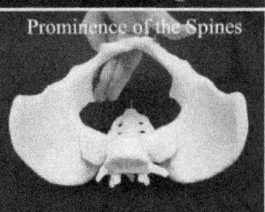

Outlet: Subpubic arch by P.V. → (≥ 90° is adequate) & (< 90° is narrow)..

Intertuberous (by external palpation) → fist on perineum, if it passing between the 2 ischial tuberosity that means it is adequate..

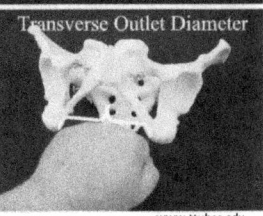

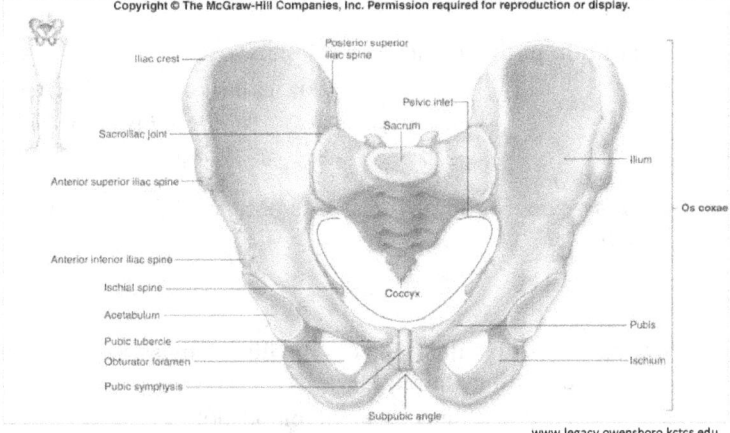

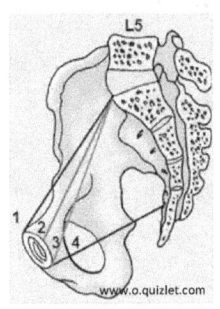

1. Anatomical conjugate - tip of the sacral promontory to the upper border of the symphysis pubis
2. Obstetrical conjugate (true conjugate) - from tip of sacral promontory to the most bulging point on the back of symphpysis pubis (about 1 cm below its upper border)
3. Diagonal conjugate (because true conjugate can't be measured) – estimated 1.5cm longer than true conjugate. From tip of sacral promontory to the lower border of the symphysis pubis. Can be measured through the vagina.
4. Straight conjugate (shortest distance) lower border of symphysis to lower border of sacrumsymphysis to lower border of sacrum

6- GYNE. & OBSTETRICS   EXAMINATION..

Post operative assessment:

HISTORY: Emergency or elective surgery ?
Date & Time of operation..

Wake up after G.A. with no problems?!!
Vomiting..
Pass urine, flatus or feces..
Movement after operation..

Fever, bleeding, pain or shortness of breath..

Start to eat ? solid or fluid ?

Any catheter ?, received blood? or take any drugs ?

In C/S → condition of child (term, pre- or post term)..
previous C/S or previous abortion..
previous uterine surgery..

Past medical & past surgical H_x ..etc

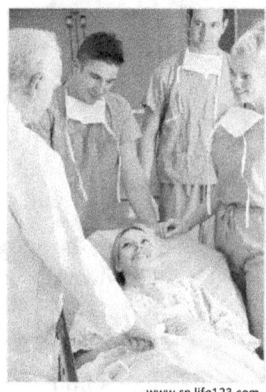
www.sp.life123.com

EXAMINATION: It is the same as what I describe in the CHAPTER ' 3 '.. But here, you have to concentrate on the following:

Palpation of the uterus → involution?
Soft or hard (normally rubbery)..
Central ? (*if not, think about broad ligament hematoma*)..

During examination, you have to observe if there is any bleeding or discharge..

NOTE: Normally, after delivery the fundus must be 1 finger breadth under the umbilicus..
If not, think about → blood clot,
full bladder or rectum,
retained piece,
infection or
fibroid..

& this is called ' *Sub-involution* '..

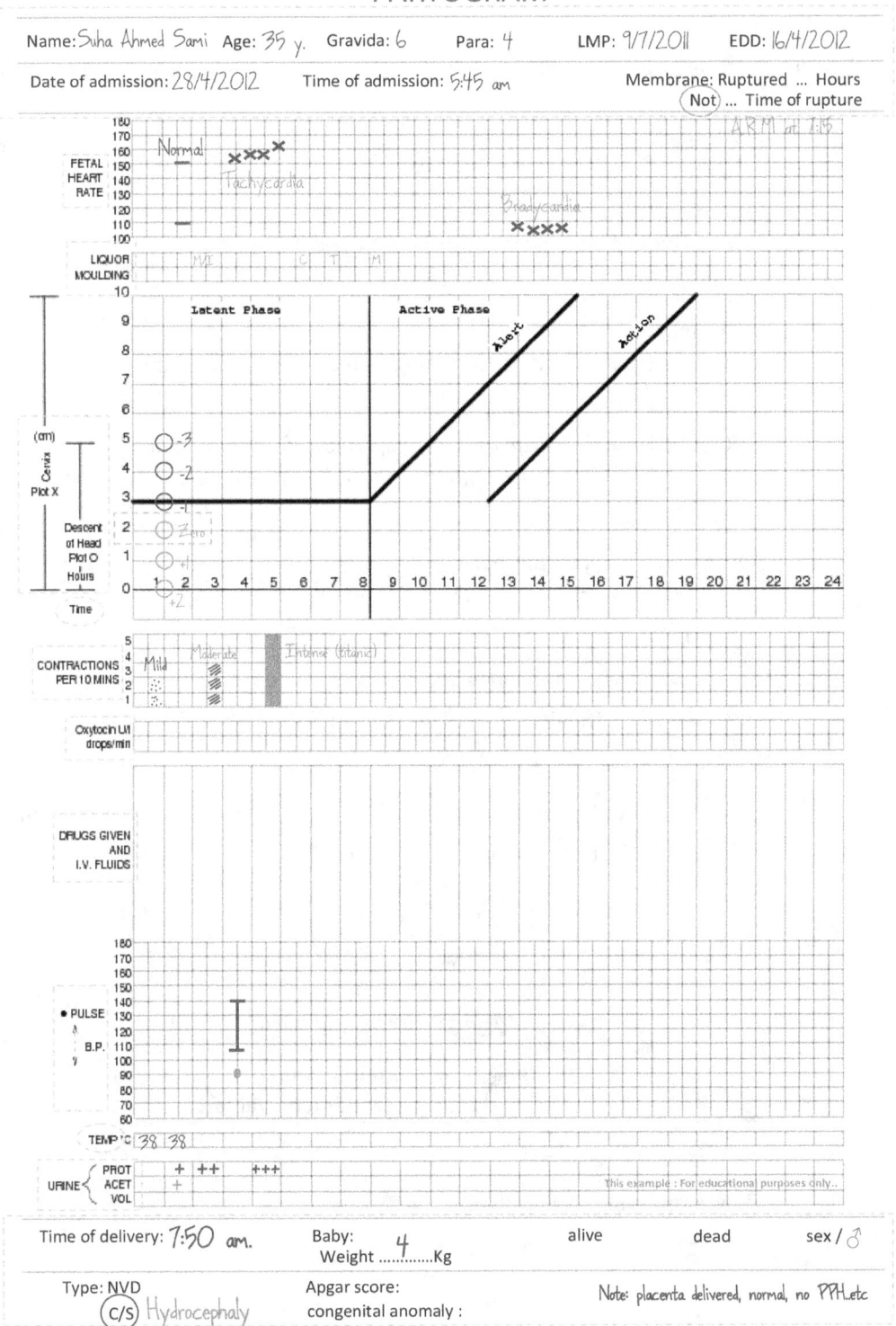

6- GYNE. & OBSTETRICS PARTOGRAM..

Partogram:

Is a graphic record of labor to illustrate the fetal & mother states, which is plotted against time in hours..

PARTOGRAM DIVISIONS: '*please, see the previous page..*'

Fetal heart rate: normal (110 -150 b.p.m.)..
abnormal either tachycardia or bradycardia..

Liquor: Intact membrane → M/I
Ruptured membrane → M/R → clear (C), thick (T) or meconium stain (M)..

Membrane: Ruptured or not + hours (if it was ruptured before admission) or
+ Time (for artificial ruptured membrane ' A.R.M. ')..

Moulding: Overlap of the fetal skull bones:
(-) → no overlap ' separated & the sutures felt easily ',
(+) → simple ' the skull bones just touch each other ',
(++) → easy ' overlapped ',
(+++) → difficult ' severely overlapped '..

Contractions / 10 mins: Must be efficient (3-4 contractions / 10 mins. *intensify* with time)..

No. of ☐ = no. of contractions..

Intensity → ⋮⋮⋮ mild (< 20 sec.),

▨ moderate (20 -40 sec.),

■ intense ' **stony hard** ' (40 -60 sec.)..

NOTE: If there are 5 **intense** contractions each (45 -60 sec)
→ there is a risk of uterus rupture..

Oxytocin: U/L & drops / min → like 30 drops /min. or
like 8 U / pint (1/2 L)..

6- GYNE. & OBSTETRICS   PARTOGRAM..

Drugs given & I.V. fluids: **any fluid, blood ..etc.**

Pulse & B.P.: *(for the mother)..*

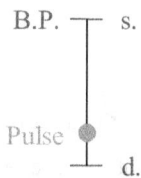

Temperature: *(for the mother)..*

Urine: Protein → P.E.
Acetone → dehydration, P.E. & D.K.A.
Volume..

Time: one **large square** → *1h.* & 1 **small square** → *1/2 h...*

Oxytocin: U/L & drops / min → like 30 drops /min. or
like 8 U / *pint* (1/2 L)..

Cervix (cm.): X → cervical dilatation…
Descent of the head: ◯ → station…

5ᵗʰ (abdominally)	Vs.	Stations (vaginally)
5		-3
4		-2
3		-1
2		0 (engagement)
1		+1
0		+2
		+3

ABNORMALITY IN CERVICAL DILATATION:

- Prolonged latent phase of 1st stage of labor..
- 1° dysfunctional labor..
- 2° arrest in 1st stage..
- 2° arrest in 2nd stage..

NOTE: Between the alert line & the action line → 4 hours..

When the cervical dilatation reaches *4 cm.* → *shift* from alert to active line..

Prolonged latent phase of 1st stage of labor:

Like: 1 cm. only every 4 h..
M$_x$: Reassurance, analgesia & mobilization ..etc

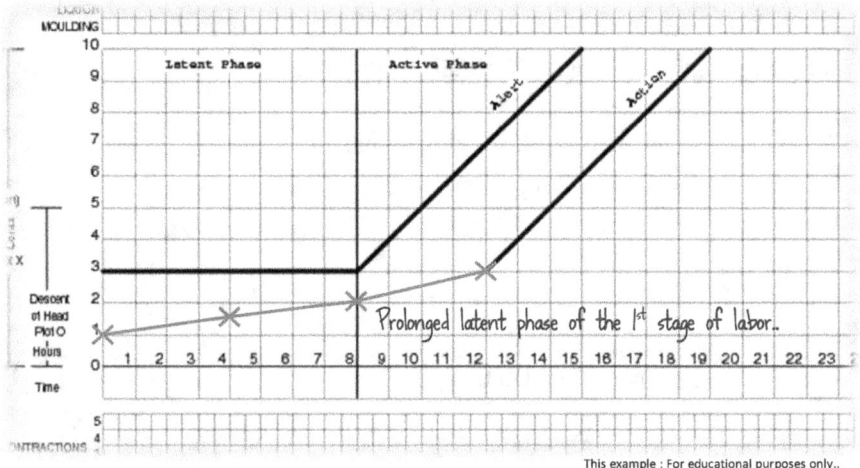

This example : For educational purposes only..

1° dysfunctional labor: ' poor progress in 1st stage before 7 cm. '..

Like: 5 cm. (after 3 h.) →6 cm. (after 4 h.) →7 cm.

Normally: 1 cm / 1h in primi.. , 2 cm. / h. in multipara..

M$_x$: Most common cause of 1° uterine dysfunction is…
    inefficient uterine contractions or irregular contractions..

So, give:
    added time &
    pain killer..

NOTE: ' After the ACTION line, you have to do an ACTION '..

So, Give analgesia..

One to one care..

If the membrane is not ruptured, yet.. Do artificial rupture membrane (A.R.M.).. Then give Oxytocin after 1/2 h..

If there is no benefit, then do → C/S..

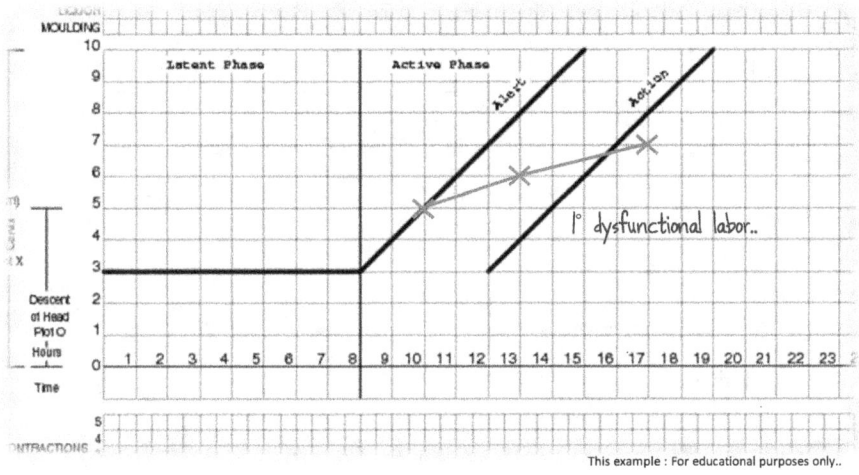

This example : For educational purposes only..

2° arrest in 1st stage of labor:

Like: 3 cm.   (after 4 h.) →6 cm.   (after 4 h.) →7 cm.   (after 4 h.) →7 cm...etc

M_x: Raise the suspension of cephalopelvic disproportion (C.P.D.)..

So, the 1st step is → *Re-evaluation..*

Big baby ?, position of the baby ?

The fifth palpable (abdominally) ?,

Breech ?

Membrane ?, moulding ?,

Do pelvimetry again..

If all are normal, but occiput transverse (mal-position) → you can give oxytocin with precaution..

Otherwise, big baby or not adequate cervix ..etc then do → C/S..

[Please see the figure in the next page..]

6- GYNE. & OBSTETRICS   PARTOGRAM..

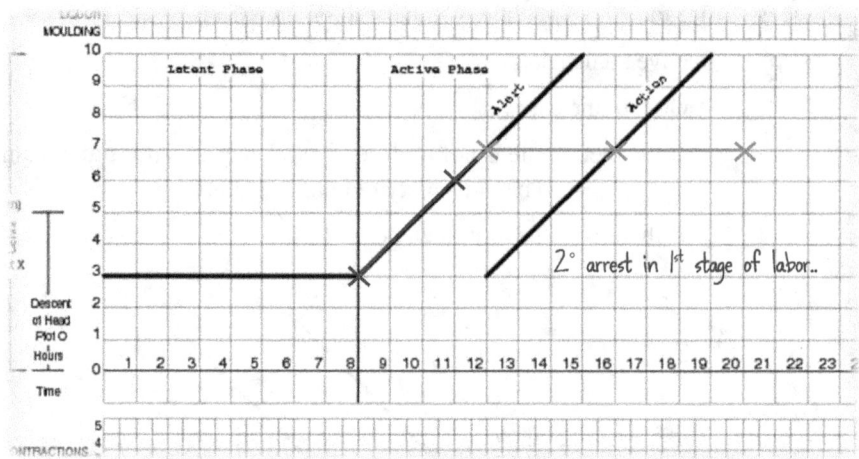

This example : For educational purposes only..

2° arrest in 2ⁿᵈ stage of labor:

    Like: $3/5^{th}$ → $3/5^{th}$ → $3/5^{th}$ (*-1 → -1 → -1 station*)..

    This may indicate C.P.D..

M_x: -1 ($3/5^{th}$) or zero ($2/5^{th}$) station → C/S is a must..

    +1 or +2 station → assisted vaginal delivery (ventose or forcepce)..

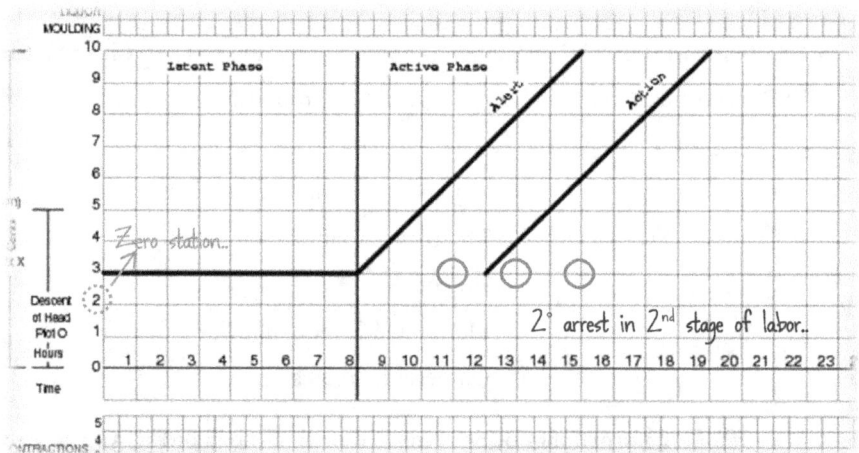

This example : For educational purposes only..

6- GYNE. & OBSTETRICS — PARTOGRAM..

IMPORTANT CASES:

- Failure to progress (ex.: 1° dysfunctional labor)..
- Chrioamnionitis..
- Fetal distress..
- Pre-eclamsia..
- Hydrocephaly..
- Cord prolapse..
- Normal labor..

Chorioamnionitis:

[Ruptured membrane > 18 h. + tachycardia + fever > 38 °C]..

M_x: Delivery (induction or C/S ..etc)..

Pre-eclamsia:

[Hypertension + proteinuria]..

Fetal distress:

[Fetal heart rate → bradycardia or tachycardia]..

M_x: Left lateral position, O_2, stop oxytocin, good hydration,

P.V. to exclude cord prolapsed & observe amniotic fluid,

Tocolytic drug → if the distress persist > 30 mins., then
do fetal scalp pH → if < 7.2 (acidosis)
then → do C/S..

Hydrocephaly:

[There is a good progress of cervical dilatation, but with **no** head descend]..

RISK FACTORS IN THE PARTOGRAM:

Age, G:P:A, EDD (so, it is important to compare it with the date of admission),

ruptured membrane & its duration, fever, proteinuria, tachycardia & hypertension..

6- GYNE. & OBSTETRICS — FORCEPS & INSTRUMENTS..

Forceps ' Short notes ':

Each forceps consists of 2 matched parts articulate together.. & each part composed of the following:
- Blade
- Shank
- Lock (English or sliding type)
- Handle

And each blade posses 2 curves:
- Cephalic curve &
- Pelvic curves..

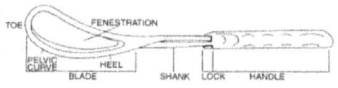
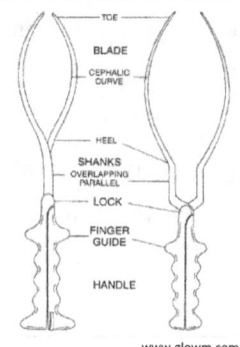

Examples:

Simpson forceps:
Used for delivery of the head while it is in the pelvis (station +2 , not engaged)..
Used for traction only..

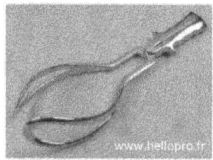

Wrigley forceps:
Used for traction of the head when the scalp visible at introitus without separation of the labia.. and fetal scull has reached pelvic floor..

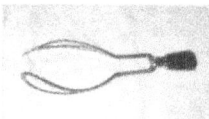

Kjelland forceps:
Rotation + traction (allow accurate cephalic application).. without separation of the labia.. and fetal scull has reached pelvic floor..
No pelvic curve in this type of forceps..

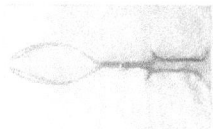

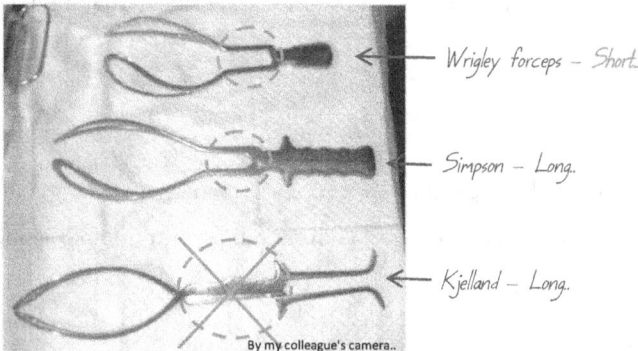

- Wrigley forceps – Short.
- Simpson – Long.
- Kjelland – Long.

Indication for assisted vaginal delivery [in general]:

- Delay in 2nd stage of labor..
- Delivery of after coming head in mal-presentation..
- Fetal distress..
- Maternal distress..

Contraindication for forceps delivery:

- Head not fully engaged..
- Cervix not fully dilated..

Complication of forceps delivery:

To the **mother:**

- Laceration of vagina, cervix or perineum..
- P.P.H..
- genital infection..

To the **infant:**

- Intracranial hemorrhage..
- Cephalohematoma..
- Facial palsy..

Indication for forceps rather than ventouse:

- Face presentation..
- Bleeding from fetal blood sampling site..
- After coming head of breach..
- delivery before 34 weeks of gestation..

Ventouse ' Short notes ':

Indication:

- Delay in 2nd stage of labor..
- Delivery of after coming head..
- Fetal distress..
- Maternal distress..

Contraindication:

- Face presentation..
- Bleeding from fetal blood sampling site..
- After coming head of breach..
- delivery before 34 weeks of gestation..

Complication:

- Genital tract trauma..
- Cervix injury..
- Chingnon..
- Cephalohematoma..
- Intracranial injury..

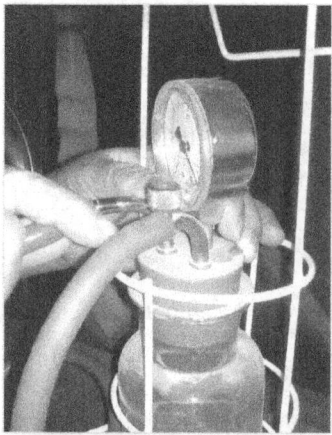
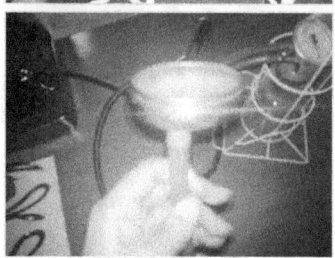

By my colleague's camera..

Instruments 'Short notes':

Sim's speculum:

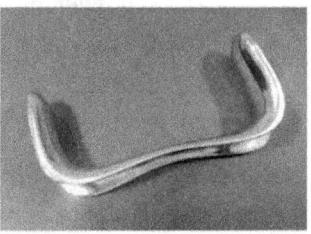

- It is non-retaining type of speculum..
- Assistant is required to hold it in position..
- The patient is put in the lithitomy position..
- The assistant hold the lower end of speculum properly for retracting the posterior vaginal wall..

  It is introduced along its edge with its blade lying vertically in anteroposterior diameter of vagina..

  Then rotate it into its position after introduction..

- **Disadvantages:** an assistant is required..
  an anterior vaginal retractor is required to get a good view..
- **Uses:** For retracting the posterior vaginal wall during:

  Dilatation & curettage (D. & C.)..
  Dilatation & evacuation (D. & E.)..
  For taking biopsy from genital tract..
  Outdoor cauterization of erosion..
  For routine per speculum examination in O.P.D..

Fergusson's speculum:

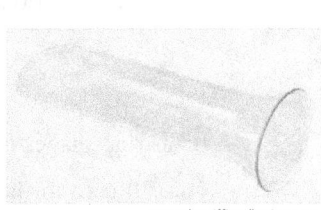

- It is a tubular speculum having no valves..
- **advantages:** It is protect the vaginal wall when it use..
- **Uses:** Taking biopsy or smear from the cervix..
  For cauterization of cervical erosions..
  For schiller's test..
  To protect the vaginal walls during decapitation operation with Gigli's wire saw..

6- GYNE. & OBSTETRICS — FORCEPS & INSTRUMENTS..

Cusco's bivalved speculum:

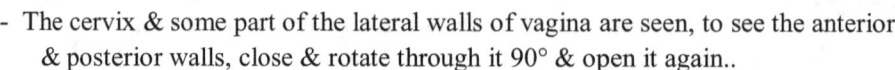

- It is self retaining type of speculum..
- It has 2 hinged blades which can be opened up & adjusted at various angles by means of screw arrangement..
- It is possible to show the cervix by this instrument..
- It is introduced into the vagina with its blades closed..
- The cervix & some part of the lateral walls of vagina are seen, to see the anterior & posterior walls, close & rotate through it 90° & open it again..
- **Advantages:** Being a self retaining speculum..
  It is easy to use..
  The vaginal walls can be retracted to a variable extent..
  It gives a good exposure of the cervix..
  Both anterior & posterior vaginal walls can be retracted with a single instrument..
  It causes least discomfort to the patient..
- **Disadvantages:** The space available for carrying out any procedure is limited by the rim of instrument..
- **Uses:** When the biopsy is to be taken from cervix..
  For cauterization of cervical erosions..
  For insertion of I.U.C.D..

Sponge (swab) holding forceps:

- It has ring shapes tips, which may be serrated or smooth..
- **Uses:** It used for holding the sponges to swab out cavities, e.g: vagina..
  Sometimes, when the anterior lip of the cervix is friable & cannot be held by volsellum, sponge holding forceps can be used..
  It can be used in place of ovum forceps..
  For applying antiseptics over vulva, vagina or abdominal skin before operation..
  It may be applied on infundibulopelvic ligaments to control bleeding in myomectomy..

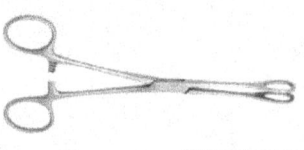

6- GYNE. & OBSTETRICS — FORCEPS & INSTRUMENTS.

Cervical dilator:
- **Types:** Hegar's dilators.
  Hawkins Ambler's dilator.
- **Uses:** Dilatation & curettage (D. & C.).
  Dilatation & evacuation (D. & E.).
  To diagnose incompetence os of cervix by passing no. 8 Hegar's dilator in non gravid uterus.
  In operations of cervix, eg: amputation of cervix, repair & cauterization of cervix.
  For insufflations tests.
  To relive some cases of spasmodic dysmenorrheal.
- **Complications:** Sepsis.
  Hemorrhage.
  Perforation of the uterus.
  Cervical tears which cause cervical incompetence or cervical dystocia at a later date.

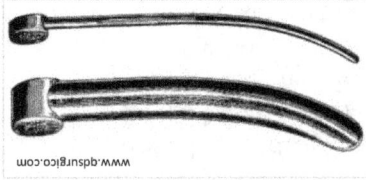
Hawkins Ambler's dilators.

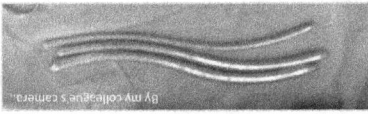
Hegar's dilators.

Anterior vaginal wall retractor:
- It has 2 loop-shaped ends with transverse serrations.
- **Uses:** It used with Sim's speculum to retract the anterior vaginal wall for visualizing the cervix & anterior fornix.

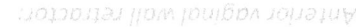

Gelpi's vulva retractors:
- This is a self retaining retractor for vulva.
- After the patient is anesthetized, this is applied to the inner walls of the vulva & opened. It is self retaining type of retractors & gives a clear opening into the vagina.

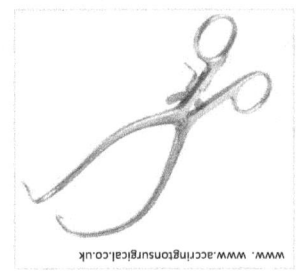

6- GYNAE. & OBSTETRICS   FORCEPS & INSTRUMENTS..

Simpson's uterine sound:

- It is a granulated metallic rod about 12 inches long..
- The distal end is curved at an angle of 60° & is 2 inches long (normal cervaical length), & the tip of the instrument is blunt..
- **Uses:** To ascertain the size & direction of the uterus before passing the cervical dilator.
  To ascertain the position of abnormal uterine contents like tumor, polyp, ..etc
  For correction of the a mobile retroverted uterus (with precaution)..
  For insufflations tests..
  The uterus is sounded routinely before operations on uterus or cervix..
- **It is not used when:** Pregnancy is suspected..
  Cervical infection is present..
- **Complications:** Sepsis..
  Perforation of the uterus..

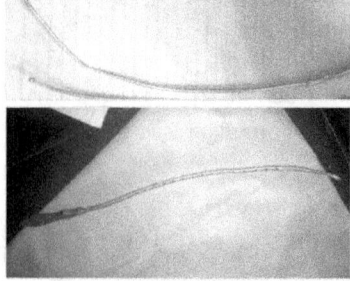

By my colleague's camera..

Bladder sound:

- It is a metallic rod, 10 inches long. It is differentiated from uterine sound by the following features.
  The curve at the distal end is uniform..
  It is not graduated..
- **Uses:** To determine the limits of the bladder during operations involving anterior vaginal wall, e.g: repair of cystocele..
  To diagnose a calculus in the bladder..
  To determine the position of urinary fistula in vagina..

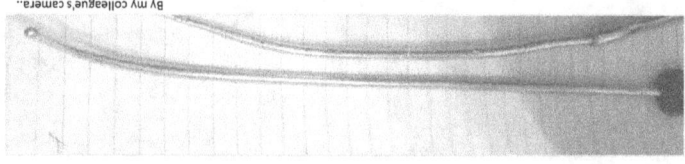

By my colleague's camera..

Uterine curettes:

- **Types:** Sim's curette..
  Goldstein curette: *(nowadays, it is not used due to the risk of fluid embolism)..*
  Sharp & blunt curette: **It is Used:**
  To curette out the products of conception in cases of missed or incomplete conception..
  To curette out endometrium in cases of endometrial diseases for diagnostic & therapeutic purposes, e.g: in cases of infertility, postmenopausal bleeding or endometrial carcinoma..
  For checking curettage done 1 w. after evacuation of hydatitiform mole..

- **Complications:** Hemorrhage..
  Sepsis..
  Perforation of the uterus..
  Vigorous curettage leads to amenorrhea due to total removal of endometrium (Asherman's syndrome)..

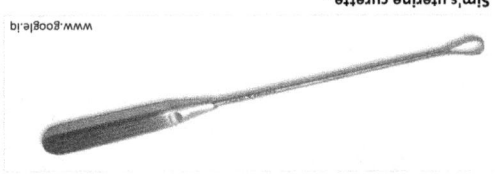

Sim's uterine curette..

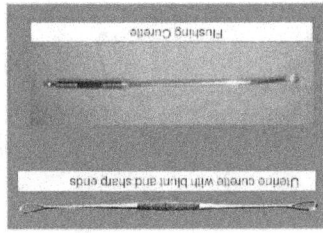

Curettes..

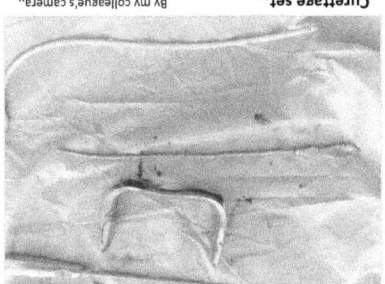

Curettage set..

Ayre's spatula:

- It is used to perform cervical smear (*pap smear*)..
- Collect the exfoliated cervical cells by a this spatula, then spread on a glass & fixed in alcohol + stain by of special stain called pap stain..
- It has (pap smear) 50% sensitivity & it is used as a screening test for cervical cancer.
- The scraping from the mucoepithelial junction (*the transitional zone*)..
- Normal cells: have small nuclei that are flattened & pyknotic while dysplastic epithelium have large nuclei, large degree of cytological atypia & high N/C ratio..
- Ideally, all women with abnormal cervical cytology should have colposcopic assessment..

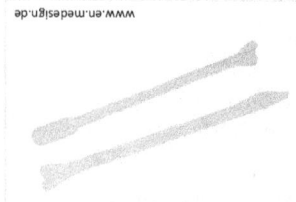

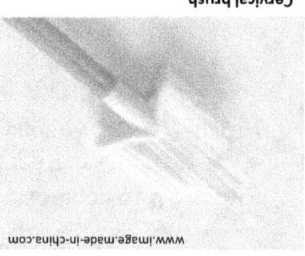

Cervical brush..

Auvard's speculum:

- It is retaining type of speculum.
- It is provided with a suitable curvature to retract the posterior vaginal wall.
- The patient is put in the lithotomy position..
- **Uses:** It is used in:
    - Major vaginal operations..
    - Amputation of the cervix in cervical cancer.
    - For repair of fistula..

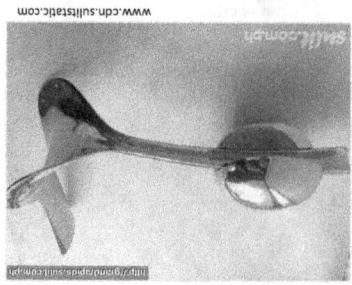

6- GYNE & OBSTETRICS — FORCEPS & INSTRUMENTS..

Volsellum forceps:

- It is used to hold the anterior lip of the cervix when it is not friable that is in gynecological conditions..
- It has got sharp teeth at the end which provide firm grip..
- **Uses:** For holding the anterior or posterior lip of cervix in various operations, e.g.: D & C, cauterization of cervix..
  To test mobility of cervix & laxity of ligaments in prolapse..
  To bring down fundus of uterus in vaginal hysterectomy.
  For small fibroids in myomectomy..

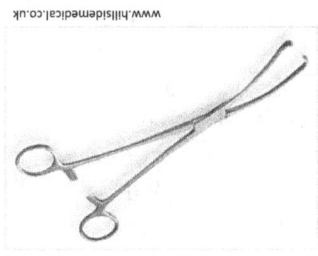

Tenaculum:

- It is simple toothed volsellum forceps & is used as volsellum..
- The advantage is that it olnly pierces the tissue at one Point, so there is very little bleeding if any..

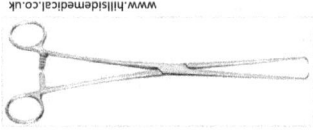

Cervical punch biopsy forceps:

- Its punched ends have a basket to hold the specimen firmly..
- It used to remove a piece from a suspicious area on cervix histopathological examination..
- If profuse bleeding occurs from the biopsied area it can be stopped by putting mattress suture..

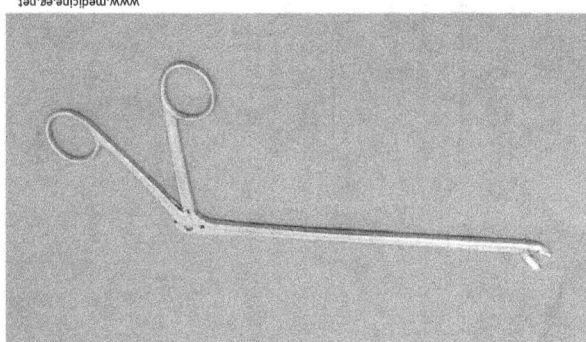

6- GYNE. & OBSTETRICS   FORCEPS & INSTRUMENTS..

Endometrial biopsy curette (Novak curette):

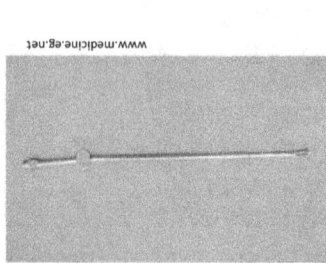

- This is a slender, hallow, blunt tipped instrument..
- It has got a notch with a cutting edge near the blunt tip..
- There is a slight angulation about 5 cm. from the tip for easier negotiation of the instrument into the uterus...
- This instrument has a stillete for removing the biopsied tissue...
- **Procedure:** The patient is put under general anesthesia or a cervical block with a sedative given prior to operation may suffice. A P.V. examination is done to determine the size & direction of the uterus, A sound is passed to confirm the length & direction. A small dilator may be used if required. Usually the curette can be passed straight away. A specimen of the cervical canal or the endometrium is then obtained...
- **Uses:** It is used in operation of fractional curettage..
  For obtaining an endometrial biopsy as in cases of T.B. uterus..
  To confirm malignancy..
  In cases of infertility to confirm the act of ovulation...

Pelvimeter:

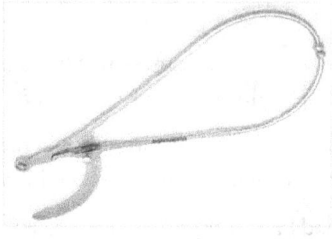

Pinard's fetoscope:

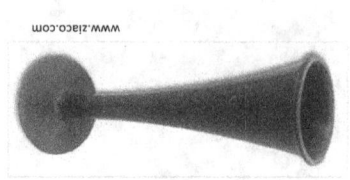

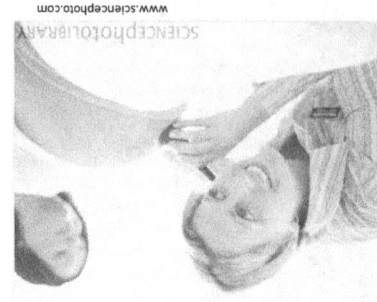

OXYTOCIN (SYNTOCINON):

Secreted from posterior part of pituitary gland & act on:

Myometrium → Cause labor (activate G protein which increase intracellular calcium level in uterine myofibrils & increase prostaglandin that stimulate uterine contraction)

Breast → cause milk secretion

Uses:
Active Mx of 3rd stage of labor (10 i.u. I.M)
Post-partum hemorrhage (40 i.u. I.M.)
Induction or augmentation of labor (ex. 8 i.u in 1 pint of N/S → 15 drops / min)
Incomplete or missed miscarriage
After molar pregnancy

Complications:
Uterine rupture
PPH
Volume overload
Fetal distress

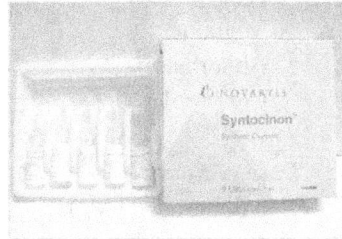

Contraindications:
CPD (cephalo-pelvic disproportion)
Previous classical scar or previous multiple scars
Fetal distress
Hypertonic uterus
Abnormal presentation (brow or shoulder)
Hypersensitivity

Rout:
I.V. & I.M

METHERGINE :

Uses :
3rd stage of labor
PPH (post-partum hemorrhage)

Complications :
Fetal distress
Uterine rupture
Hypertension
Retained placenta

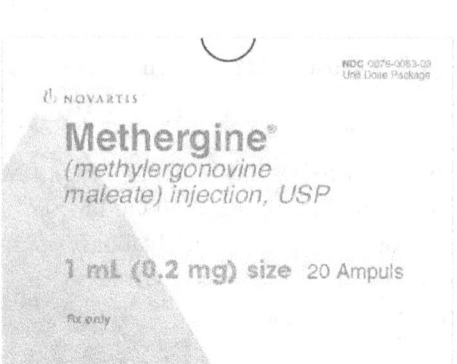

Contraindications :
Hypertension
Heart disease
Migraine
Abnormal lie
Cord prolapse

Dose & Rout : :
0.5 mg/ml (I.V.)